Intermittent Fasting

for Women Over 50 in Menopause

Powerful Protocols for Losing Weight, Boosting Metabolism, Feeling Healthier and Happier Through All Stages

Table of Contents

Introduction: Fasting, Menopause, and You 7

Chapter 1: Everything You Need to Know 9

Intermittent Fasting 101: Your One-Stop Knowledge Shop 9

Intermittent Fasting: What Happens to the Body? 11

Brain Health and Aging 11

Human Growth Hormone (HGH) 12

Insulin Levels 13

Cellular Repair 13

Gene Expression 14

Inflammation 14

Heart Health 15

Cancer 15

Musculoskeletal Health 16

Weight Loss & Menopause: The Resounding Question 16

How It's Done 18

Meal Skipping: The One You Don't Think About 19

The Twelve-Hour Method: Half A Day 19

A Sixteen Hour Fast: The Nitty Gritty 20

The 18:6 Method: The Intermediate Fast 20

Warrior Method: An Advanced Fast 20

Alternate Day Fasting: Switch It Up 21

Two-Day Fast: The 5:2 Diet 21

24-Hour Fast: A Once-a-Week Option 22

It's Your Choice 22

Potential Side-Effects: Why They Happen & What to Do 23

Cravings 23

Lightheadedness 23

Digestive Issues 23

Irritability & Frustration 24

Sleep Disturbances 24

Bad Breath 24

Mild Dehydration 25

Your Fasting Journey: Revamp Your Mindset 25

Chapter 2: Changing Your Mind 26

Is It Time to Cleanse? 27

The Physical: Is Your Body Telling You to Cleanse? 27

The Brain: Is It Telling You It's Time?..29

The Spiritual: Are You in Touch With Yourself?..31

Don't Overdo It..32

So Why Cleanse? What Do I Get Out Of It?..33

Fasting & Cleansing the Brain..33

Fasting & Brain Cells..33

Cognition and Mood..34

Mental Disease and Decline...34

Fasting and Mental Health..35

Fasting, Cleansing, and Metabolism: The Be-All Breakdown...35

Preparing for a Fast..36

Drink Fluids...36

Think About How You'll Break Your Fast...37

Pay Attention & Adjust..37

What to Expect Hour by Hour...38

Listening to Your Body: How to Move Forward..39

Chapter 3: A History of Intermittent Fasting...41

Diet Culture: The Weird, the Odd, and the Crazy...42

A History of Intermittent Fasting: Stepping Back in Time...43

Intermittent Fasting in Ancient Times...43

Fasting as Holistic Medicine: Healing Your Body & Soul...46

Our Modern Relationship With Food...47

Back to Basics: Reviving the Practice..48

Chapter 4: The Unspoken Secrets of Success...49

Common Mistakes & Misconceptions...50

You Don't Ease Into It..51

You're Consuming Too Many Calories..51

You're Sabotaging With Soda..52

You Aren't Drinking Enough..53

You're Not Eating the Right "Fast-Breaking" Foods..53

Your Approach Was Too Extreme..54

You're Going Through Caffeine Withdrawals...55

You Work Out Too Hard...55

You're Overthinking...56

You Give Up Altogether...56

Keeping Yourself Full: Food & Drinks..57

Your Fasting Drink Guide...57

Water, Tea, and Coffee: The Starter Pack..58

Apple Cider Vinegar & Bone Broth: Best Kept Secrets...59

Salt: The Spice That (May or May Not) Make Everything Nice 59

Your Go-to Food Guide **60**

To Eat or Not to Eat: The Menopause Question 60

Menopause, Hot Flashes, and Food: What Gives? 63

The Power of Protein 63

Sleep: The Biggest Secret 66

Misconceptions Aside: What Comes Next? **71**

Chapter 5: Move More **73**

Should I Exercise? **74**

Working Out While Fasting: Disclaimers and Notes 76

Why It May Not Be Effective 76

How to Do It the Right Way 76

Planning Your Routine 77

Yoga: The Faster's Crash Course **79**

Improved Strength and Balance 80

Improved Flexibility 80

Yoga and Heart Health 81

Trouble Falling Asleep? Try Yoga 81

Yoga and Self-Esteem 82

Yoga and Mental Health 83

Yoga and Menopause: Why and How 83

Fun Ways to Move **87**

Move Forward **88**

Chapter 6: Perimenopause Food and Fasting Plan **89**

What Is Menopause? **89**

Perimenopause: What, Why, and Is It Happening to you? 90

The Perimenopause Diet **91**

Plant-Based Foods 92

Fiber 92

Vitamins and Minerals 93

Omega-3 Fatty Acids 95

How to Eat Like a Perimenopause Intermittent Fasting Pro **95**

Breakfast 96

Lunch 101

Dinner 106

Snacks 112

Perimenopause Cooking: Key Takeaways **117**

Chapter 7: Mid-Menopause **118**

What Is Mid-Menopause? **118**

The Mid-Menopause Diet...119

    Dairy Products...119

    Whole Grains..120

    Phytoestrogens...120

The Mid-Menopause Healthy Meal Plan......................................120

    Breakfast...122

    Lunch...127

    Dinner..132

    Snacks...137

Food Is The Cure: Mid-Menopause Diet......................................141

Chapter 8: Post-Menopause..142

What Is Post-Menopause?...142

Concerns During Post-Menopause...143

What to Eat..144

    Vitamin C Rich Foods...144

    Dietary Phytoestrogens..144

    Unsaturated Fats...144

    Calcium..145

    Vitamin D...145

Five-Day Post-Menopause Food Plan..146

    Breakfast...147

    Lunch...152

    Dinner..157

    Snacks...162

Your Post-Menopausal Future..167

Conclusion: Don't Fear the Future...168

References..171

Introduction:

Fasting, Menopause, and You

"Women are like teabags. We don't know our strength until we are in hot water."

- Eleanor Roosevelt

I entered menopause when I was about 48. If you're familiar with menopause, you know this firsthand—it sucks, regardless of age, circumstances, or environment.

I felt confused, and, for the lack of a better word, angry. I had the Internet, so I dove into Google, Reddit, and Quora searches for answers to my never-ending list of questions.

"How long should hot flashes last?"

"Should I be breaking out?"

"Why am I gaining weight?"

"Menopause neck pain?"

These are just a few of what I'd assume was thousands of searches I did while trying to navigate my changing body.

My symptoms were nothing unusual: hot flashes, fatigue, headaches, waking up in the middle of the night drenched in sticky sweat, etc. But, to me, they were completely foreign. What was happening to me?

Menopause is scary. It's not a living room or dinner party topic. It's a little like the birds and the bee's conversation you had with your parents—they spoke in hushed tones behind closed doors about taboo topics.

Because of this, it's hard to get real, reliable information from the source.

You're not alone. For me, menopause didn't hit me until I began feeling its physical effects like bloating, mood changes, and shifting perceived body image issues. Most women feel similarly—body image seems like the first thing out the window during perimenopause.

91% of women across all age groups feel a degree of dissatisfaction with their bodies, and we can assume the number is higher for women entering menopause. Menopausal weight gain is common, but it comes as a real dismay for many women.

If you're feeling frustrated, angry, bitter, or experiencing the full-fledged symptoms of menopause, you're in good company.

I felt similarly.

I'd been practicing intermittent fasting on and off since my early twenties. My fasting journey wasn't initially intentional, but, over time, I loved what it did to my body. I felt clear, calm, and logical—not to mention what happened to my waistline!

I gave up on intermittent fasting in my early forties. Life gets complicated: work, family, chores, and engagements get in the way, and I let my health fall by the wayside.

It wasn't until I researched intermittent fasting and menopause symptom relief that I felt I'd cracked the code.

I felt more energized, lost a little bit of weight, and felt much healthier. It doesn't happen overnight; it might take a while.

But this isn't about me; this is about you and your mental, physical, and spiritual health.

Chapter 1:
Everything You Need to Know

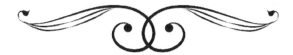

"I'm interested in women's health because I'm a woman.
I'd be a darn fool not to be on my own side."

– Maya Angelou

Welcome to your intermittent fasting crash course! In this Chapter, I'll provide all the information you need about why, how, and what to watch out for when beginning your intermittent fasting journey and how it relates to menopause symptoms.

Keep in mind that there is no "one size fits all" fast. Everybody is different, and it's okay to make modifications to a certain fasting method, especially while you're getting started.

Your body might need more time to adapt than you thought, and that's okay.

Listen to your body throughout the entire process. Think about what you're feeling at this moment. Use this Chapter to decide which method is right for you.

Intermittent Fasting 101: Your One-Stop Knowledge Shop

Intermittent fasting involves alternating between periods of fasting and periods of normal eating. The length of these periods varies depending on your preferences; some prefer to participate in a longer fast, between sixteen and twenty-four hours, while others do a shorter, more "incidental" fast, but I'll discuss these methods in more depth later in this chapter.

Always consult your doctor before beginning a fast. You come first.

Most diets dictate you eat certain foods. Those practicing the keto diet can't eat carbohydrates and rely on meat products, certain vegetables, and carbohydrate-friendly dairy products to hit their nutrient goals. Those trying the Mediterranean diet eat lean meats, seafood, whole wheat products, etc.

Fasting is different. Fasting "doesn't specify which foods you should eat but rather when you should eat them," which is relatively unheard of within the diet and wellness community (Gunners, 2020).

When practicing fasting, you don't restrict what you eat, though eating a healthy, colorful, protein-rich diet is always important. Instead, intermittent fasters focus on *when* they eat. It's both a cost-effective (and taste-effective) way to change your body.

But that's not the only plus; you can easily meet your nutritional needs! You don't have to forego entire food groups or certain products; it's your responsibility to meet your nutritional goals and guidelines.

In many ways, fasting is a natural "diet." Many people forego breakfast or lunch anyway, so for them, it's an easy transition.

Use me as an example. I was an intermittent faster in my twenties and I didn't even know it. I worked long hours, so breakfast was normally an afterthought. I would eat dinner around 7 pm, but I ate my first meal the next day around noon.

Fasting isn't starving yourself; in fact, it's anything but. Don't go into a fasting habit with that mindset. Restriction is the most common reason why people stop dieting. Instead, listen to your body and create a plan that works for you.

Like any lifestyle change, fasting comes with its own set of pros and cons; we'll talk about it together. Let's start with the pros.

Intermittent fasting is a very simple, wallet-friendly way to lose weight and reap amazing long-term health benefits.

Not only that but there's nothing off-limits. Eating a relatively healthy diet is always recommended, but there's nothing in the research telling you that you can't indulge in the occasional chocolate bar. It's pretty flexible. You choose when you fast, how you fast, and when you exercise.

Additionally, fasting makes it easy to maintain other dietary habits, religious practices, and personal preferences. Other diets require you consume certain foods to attain certain results, which marginalizes those with dietary restrictions. You can follow the diet while remaining gluten-free, vegan, vegetarian, halal, kosher, and low-fat.

Fasting doesn't allow your body to get "used" to the change. Some fasters choose to do a prolonged 48-hour fast one week but choose to participate in a shorter-term fast the week following.

Many dieters report a weight loss plateau around the three-month mark: over time, our bodies become used to a diet, and it becomes less effective. Intermittent fasting is a cycle, so that doesn't happen.

There are a few disclaimers. Pregnant women and young children shouldn't try intermittent fasting. Additionally, those suffering from eating disorders or other mental health disorders should stay away from intermittent fasting. For those going through menopause, pregnancy might not be a concern, but if you're on the fence, consult a medical professional.

Intermittent fasting may cause fluctuations in insulin levels, so those suffering from Type 1 diabetes should take caution. However, those with Type 2 diabetes are just fine. Intermittent fasting yields incredible benefits for those with pre-diabetes or Type 2 diabetes.

If you're taking prescription medication or suffer from liver or kidney disease, take note. You can still engage in intermittent fasting, but again, consult a medical professional before making any drastic health changes.

Intermittent Fasting: What Happens to the Body?

Intermittent fasting isn't a diet. It's a wellness plan.

I'll call this the "science section," but if you weren't a biology person back in school, don't be alarmed.

I'll break it down for you.

Brain Health and Aging

Intermittent fasting changes your brain, and for the better.

Brain-derived neurotrophic factor (BDNF) is an essential protein that supports neurons in the brain; it's linked to the progression of neurodegenerative diseases like Alzheimer's, Dementia, etc.

Low levels of BDNF are thought to be partially responsible for the development of these conditions and diseases.

Intermittent fasting causes "systemic inflammation" (not the bad kind) that prevents "the reduction of BDNF levels in the hippocampus" (Francis, 2020). This is especially important; higher levels of brain-derived neurotrophic factor support memory, prevent neurodegenerative diseases, and aid in cognitive functioning.

There is a strong link between mitochondrial function and degenerative diseases; think back to high school—the mitochondria are the powerhouse of the cell! Mitochondria play an "important [role] in maintaining intracellular signaling networks that modulate various cellular functions" (Zhao et al., 2022).

But it goes a step further; researchers know that mitochondrial dysfunction is an early sign of cognitive decline in older adults. Over time, intermittent fasting improves mitochondrial functioning and can prevent the onset of Alzheimer's, Parkinson's, and Huntington's disease.

Here's the takeaway: Intermittent fasting stimulates proteins and cell function to prevent the onset of cognitive diseases.

Human Growth Hormone (HGH)

Human growth hormone, otherwise known as HGH, is produced in your pituitary gland and influences your body's metabolism, cell growth and development, and body composition. When our HCH levels are high, we become more focused and recover more quickly from disease or illness.

I'll explain. Human growth hormone plays a role in anti-aging and protects the brain against neurodegenerative diseases; it stimulates fat utilization and aids in protein conservation, which aids in muscular development, weight regulation, and prevents long-term cognitive illness.

But does HGH relate to menopause? Yes!

During menopause, estrogen levels drop as your ovaries gradually stop producing eggs. Unfortunately, HGH and estrogen go hand in hand: When estrogen levels are high, so are HGH levels. In fact, "the more estrogen a woman has, the more HGH she produces" (Gunasekara, 2019). So, when estrogen levels drop, human growth hormone levels also decline.

When HGH levels are low you'll notice more fat around your stomach, low libido, and poor skin quality, among other symptoms.

Fasting boosts human growth hormone levels, allowing us to heal, rejuvenate, and recoup. It's a key lifestyle choice for women during menopause.

Insulin Levels

Insulin is a hormone that controls and regulates blood sugar levels. When we eat a large, carbohydrate-heavy meal, our insulin levels increase to help our liver process glucose. During periods of low carbohydrate consumption or fasting, our insulin levels drop. There's no glucose to process, so your body begins burning fat.

Insulin gets a bad reputation, but it's important.

The hormone becomes an issue when we develop insulin resistance. When our bodies become insulin-resistant, our blood sugar increases. It doesn't sound too scary, but it can be. It's a balance: When we become insulin-resistant, insulin in the body can't aid in the processing of glucose, and, as a result, there's more glucose (or sugar) in places it shouldn't be.

When our blood sugar increases rapidly and often, it potentially damages nerve cells and bodily tissues. Over time, we can develop Type 2 diabetes.

But when you're going through menopause, it's an especially important consideration. During menopause, your hormone levels become a sort of roller coaster, ultimately changing the way your body uses and responds to insulin. Your insulin levels increase and decrease more readily, and these fluctuations can increase your risk of Type 2 diabetes.

Don't freak out! Fasting is here to help!

Insulin levels drop during a fast in response to the lack of glucose. Fasting gives your liver a breather. Scientists theorize that those who follow an intermittent fasting regimen experience 3-6% lower blood sugar levels than their non-fasting counterparts. I'll go into this more in the next chapter, but, as a whole, lower insulin levels prevent insulin resistance.

Cellular Repair

During a fast, our bodies begin what's called autophagy, the process by which dead or oxidized cells are removed from the body, paving the way for new cells and tissues.

It's a scary word, but there's nothing scary about it!

Studies show that intermittent fasting may cause activation of our body's "adaptive cellular stress response" and signals pathways, "that enhance mitochondrial health, DNA repair and autophagy" (Mattson et al., 2017).

Other studies show a link between immune cell health and intermittent fasting; when fasting, "old" immune cells die and are readily replaced by new stem cells, improving immune system responses.

That's a lot of science, so I'll explain it further.

We discussed mitochondria earlier in the chapter. Improving mitochondrial health enhances our health on a cellular level, triggering DNA repair processes. Pretty cool, right?

Gene Expression

Intermittent fasting may play a role in gene expression, or the way genes are physically expressed in our appearance, or mechanically expressed in bodily functions.

It sounds a little odd, but it's science.

Studies show that those practicing intermittent fasting experience changes in the way their genetics are expressed, especially those that code for anti-aging proteins. You buy anti-aging skin serums, creams, and products at the store; why not try something similar for your body?

Inflammation

No one enjoys feeling bloated. But bloating, otherwise known as chronic inflammation, goes beyond the feeling you experience when you try on your favorite jeans and they don't fit quite right. Chronic inflammation can lead to long-term disease.

Unfortunately, bloating is a common side effect of menopause, especially in perimenopause and mid-menopause. As estrogen and progesterone levels destabilize, your body begins to hold onto water in unwanted places.

However, fasting can help.

Bloating is often a sign your digestive system is out of wack; your body is telling you that water, essential nutrients, and minerals aren't being digested properly, and these irregularities cause bloating.

The number of monocytes, cells responsible for inflammation in the body, drops during periods of fasting. Scientists aren't sure why, but it's something to keep in mind. Many scientists and prominent physicians prescribe fasting for those suffering from bloating.

You might notice a little more bloating than usual when you begin a fast. Your body needs a little time to get used to your new lifestyle. As your body adapts to a consistent fasting routine, you'll notice less inflammation in your legs, upper arms, and stomach area.

Heart Health

Most people take great measures to care for their heart; we do cardio-based workouts, eat heart-healthy foods, and abstain from smoking.

But it's not just about your heart. It's about what goes through it.

There are two types of cholesterol: LDL, or "bad" cholesterol, and HDL, or "good" cholesterol. LDL cholesterol can deposit within your arterial walls over time, especially if you're genetically predisposed to heart disease.

This cholesterol or plaque builds up, leading to inflammation and heart disease.

Plaque buildup isn't the only thing increasing your risk for heart disease: Doctors report that, after menopause, a woman's risk of a heart attack greatly increases.

Keep in mind that menopause doesn't necessarily cause heart disease, but some menopausal symptoms, like cravings, can increase your risk.

But again, fasting is a solution.

Fasting changes the way your body metabolizes food. It's thought these changes lead to lower levels of LDL cholesterol. When our bodies distribute fat in a healthy way, our heart responds positively.

Cancer

Dead and oxidized cells are primarily responsible for certain cancers. During a fast, our bodies go through autophagy, or the removal and disposal of these cells, leading to a lower incidence of certain cancers.

A woman's risk of cancer increases after menopause. Hormone levels become erratic and change rapidly, confusing your body.

Studies show that late menopause increases one's risk of cancer even more. Women who go into perimenopause after age 54 have a higher risk of both breast and endometrial cancer because they've been exposed to more estrogen throughout their lives.

Recent studies point to a link between intermittent fasting and a lower rate of recurrence in breast cancer. Intermittent fasting improves metabolic health and medical professionals acknowledge that "metabolic disturbances, like too much insulin and blood sugar, increase the risk of breast cancer recurring" (Piersol, 2020).

Because of this, intermittent fasting reduces "the risk that breast cancer will come back after treatment" (Piersol, 2020).

Musculoskeletal Health

Women are more susceptible to bone diseases such as osteoporosis and arthritis. It's a fact of life. I watched my grandmother struggle with these diseases: In just a few short months, she went from a tennis-playing pro to a woman who could barely make it to the kitchen.

Intermittent fasting plays a strong role in hormone regulation and human growth hormone secretion. Certain minerals, like calcium, aid in bone health, but over time, our bodies don't absorb these minerals as readily.

One study that looked at 76 women above the age of thirty noticed that, after the fasting period, macrophage levels (responsible for aiding in muscle development) increased, suggesting a positive correlation between intermittent fasting and muscular support (Liu et al., 2019).

Intermittent fasting's effect on hormone regulation and protein development maintains important mechanisms that support long-term muscle and bone health.

In other words, intermittent fasting can help you play tennis like Serena Williams for a lifetime!

Weight Loss & Menopause: The Resounding Question

The process of menopause seems to be one of society's "best-kept" secrets. There's nothing "best" about it.

Menopause stinks; I know this firsthand. It's an unfortunate reality for women. Our bodies change and our cognitive function becomes a bit cloudy.

Here's where you come in. Let's discuss some of the changes you'll experience (or are experiencing) during menopause, and how intermittent fasting targets some of these changes.

You've likely noticed some differences in weight loss and weight gain over the past few years. Weight loss is easy in your late teens and early twenties. We can virtually look at a treadmill and lose five pounds. As we get older, weight loss is trickier.

But it's science and, contrary to what you might believe, all fat isn't the same.

Belly fat, otherwise known as the abdominal distribution of adipose tissue, is linked to a greater incidence of heart disease and diabetes as opposed to fat distributed in other areas of your body.

If you're a pear-shaped gal like me, you're in a bit of luck.

If not, that's okay too. Studies show those following an intermittent fasting regimen "lost 4–7% of their waist circumference, indicating a significant loss of harmful belly fat that builds up around your organs and causes disease" (Gunnars, 2022)

Let's take it a step further.

During menopause, you might experience cravings, which play a role in your ability to lose weight. It's frustrating. It's angering. You can go to the gym every day (though this isn't recommended) and still experience a seemingly unusual attraction to the chocolate bar sitting in your cabinet.

Menopause causes cravings that are nothing short of intrusive. Many women report that menopause cravings contribute to bodily "stress and unwanted weight gain" (Winona Editorial Team & Green, 2022).

It stinks, but it's science. Let's break it down.

When we indulge in certain foods like chocolate, salty popcorn, large ribeye steaks, or ice cream sundaes, our brains feel happy. It's a reward and a big one. Our taste buds tell our brains that these foods make us feel good because they're undeniably tasty. Our reward center lights up like a Christmas tree.

Sweet, salty, fatty, and delicious foods are called hyper-palatable foods, otherwise known as "comfort foods." Ruffles potato chips are my hyper-palatable food of choice.

When our estrogen and progesterone levels are nice and balanced, the appetite-suppressing hormone leptin makes us feel full. It's released in the right place and at the right time; it tells our brains that we're satisfied and ready to take on what's next.

Menopause throws our hormones a curveball. Estrogen and progesterone levels decrease, which contributes to the powerful cravings you experience late at night or in the afternoon. Leptin isn't released as normal and ghrelin (the hunger hormone) levels increase. You're hungry more often and you reach for a snack.

Unfortunately, that's not all. During menopause, our bodies hold onto unwanted belly fat, which only aggravates hormonal changes. Estrogen and progesterone levels drop like a rock in a well.

When we engage in intermittent fasting, we lose some of this belly fat and our hormone levels stabilize. As a result, we feel more satisfied, energized, and confident.

How It's Done

So how do you do it? Well, there are many ways we can engage in intermittent fasting. Again, intermittent fasting isn't starvation. It's anything but. We alternate between periods of restriction and periods of virtual food freedom.

You're restricting without thinking about it and that's what makes intermittent fasting different from other diets. There isn't a hard and fast rule; you don't need to go to the grocery store and stock up on wheat germ and chia seeds.

Another benefit is that you can sleep while you fast! While you're sleeping, your body rejuvenates itself to prepare you for the following day, but it goes through similar digestive processes as it would while you're awake. It does the calorie-burning for you while you're not thinking about it.

So what types of intermittent fasting methods are out there? We'll start small and then discuss the larger, more "difficult" types of intermittent fasting.

These aren't the only types of intermittent fasting out there. Some advanced fasters choose long-term water fasts to fully cleanse their bodies. These diets aren't for the faint of heart, and few existing studies are proving their efficacy. For the purposes of this book, I'll stick to scientifically proven fasting methods.

Meal Skipping: The One You Don't Think About

You don't need a timer or stopwatch for this one; it's the oldest trick in the book.

In my younger years, I would simply forget meals. I'd roll out of bed twenty minutes late and rush my way to work.

When you're in your late teens and twenties, you might forego breakfast and reach for a cup of coffee. Perhaps you forgot to pack your lunch. It's pretty common. You were engaging in intermittent fasting and you had no idea!

Meal skipping is, in my opinion, the easiest way to begin intermittent fasting. If you're not feeling too hungry one morning, skip breakfast. If you're not hungry around noon, skip lunch.

Check out the following example.

Let's say you eat a yummy dinner at 7 pm. You read a book, spend a bit of time with family, and head to bed around 10 pm. You wake up to your alarm the next morning and realize you're already late for your 9 am meeting! You take a quick rinse-off shower, pour yourself some coffee, and run to your car. Your commute is a blur and you make it to your meeting in the nick of time.

Your meeting lasts until 11 am and you grab an apple and some pretzels from the corner store around noon.

You just fasted for sixteen hours and barely thought about it. This is a relatively common practice for most Americans.

A meal-skipping fast doesn't need to be a daily practice. You might forego breakfast one day but eat pancakes and sausage the next.

It's intermittent fasting without planning.

The Twelve-Hour Method: Half A Day

This method takes a little more thought than meal skipping, but it's still pretty easy. It's just like it sounds–you fast for twelve hours!

Let's use the same example as the one before. You eat your dinner (spaghetti, meatballs, and homemade garlic bread) around 7 pm. You knit, read, or watch TV. Whatever suits your fancy. You get ready for bed around 10 pm and set your alarm for 7 am the next morning.

You wake up around seven (you're on time today) so you grab a quick bowl of cereal. You fasted for twelve hours.

A Sixteen Hour Fast: The Nitty Gritty

Here's where the water deepens. The main difference between a sixteen-hour fast and meal skipping is that, in an intentional sixteen-hour fast, you're thinking about it. It's a daily habit.

The 16:8 fasting plan is arguably the most common type of fasting. It's my method of choice. Like the others, it's relatively self-explanatory. You don't eat for sixteen hours but eat normally for eight.

As I said, it's a daily practice, but it's ultimately possible. Instead of simply forgetting your breakfast, you bring it with you to work and wait until noonish to dive in. Your meal can be virtually anything, though I'll touch on that later. You eat normally for those eight hours and go straight to bed.

The 18:6 Method: The Intermediate Fast

The 18:6 method is much like the 16:8 one, but with a more challenging twist.

Again, it's pretty self-explanatory, but I'll go into more detail for you.

The 18:6 method involves normal eating for six hours followed by an eighteen-hour fast. It's doable, but not for the faint of heart.

The easiest way to go about the 18:6 protocol is as follows.

You eat a whole grain BLT with tortilla chips and salsa for lunch at noon, followed by your snack of choice (mine is carrots and red-pepper hummus) around 2 pm. At four, you eat another, more substantial snack and, for dinner, you eat again. Business as normal.

18:6 fasters may choose not to eat anything between the hours of 6 pm and noon the following day. You might feel a little lethargic, so don't try this method first. It's intermediate for a reason.

Warrior Method: An Advanced Fast

The warrior fasting method is the most "advanced" fasting protocol before you get into longer or prolonged fasts.

The warrior diet isn't necessarily a fast in the traditional sense; instead, it's a diet plan built off traditional fasting methods.

Those following the warrior diet use a 20:4 model. However, during the twenty-hour window, you can eat small things. I mean *very* small. As in, "hard-boiled egg, a cup of coffee, a small bag of carrots" small. During the four-hour nonfasting period, you can eat whatever you'd like.

Those following the warrior diet might eat from 4 pm to 8 pm but choose a timeframe that works for you. Your nonfasting meals consist of whatever healthy options you'd like: shrimp and grits, rich tomato sauces, chocolate-covered strawberries, etc. There's no limit on the number of calories you can consume during this period. For most, it's a relatively high number.

However, during the rest of the day, those following the warrior diet eat tiny meals: handfuls of nuts, no sugar, raw vegetables, etc.

It's considered the most restrictive short-term intermittent fasting protocol, but it's nevertheless one to think about.

It's important to note that the jury is out regarding the viability of the warrior method. It's effective all right; the real question is: Is it healthy? And is it promoting a healthy attitude towards dieting? Some believe the warrior method encourages binge eating so proceed with caution.

Alternate Day Fasting: Switch It Up

The next few fasting methods I'll discuss involve a 24-hour fast; what differs is the frequency. During an alternate day fast, you simply alternate! It's not too complicated.

On one day, you'll consume around 25% of your normal caloric intake. Most people eat around 500 calories during their "fasting" day. What you decide to eat is up to you, though most alternate-day fasters choose to eat nutrient-dense foods like vegetables, nuts, protein, or fruits.

You might be tempted to indulge in your energy-dense meal of choice during your fasting day, especially after a few hours. Here's the kicker, you can't consume more than 500 or so calories. Most people want to space out their meals. If you loaded up on pretzels, you'd hit your goal in minutes. The next day, alternate day fasters eat what they'd like.

It's not too complicated.

Two-Day Fast: The 5:2 Diet

Much like the alternate day fast, the 5:2 fasting method involves eating few to no calories for two days a week, followed by five days of normal eating.

The bright side of the 5:2 method is you can choose which days work best for you!

Most following this method opt to fast during the week so they can enjoy meals with family and friends on weekends, but the choice is ultimately yours.

Some "hardcore" fasters don't eat at all during the two fasting days, while intermediate fasters eat a few healthy snacks on a fasting day. Again, it's up to you!

24-Hour Fast: A Once-a-Week Option

This one is just a variation of the others we've discussed. Instead of fasting on alternate days or for two days a week, you fast for one.

This is a great option for beginning or intermediate fasters; you're able to glean fasting's benefits without too much commitment or headache.

A 24-hour fast is particularly effective for those struggling with their schedule. We're all busy people, and a 24-hour fast is a great way to knock out your fasting routine in one fell swoop!

24-hour fasters usually choose to fast during the weekend, but others prefer to fast during the week. When you fast is up to you.

It's also permissible to change your fasting days once in a while. You might have a birthday party or family dinner on your normal fasting day and that's okay! Choose another day for your 24-hour fast.

Most fasters following the one-day fast forego food altogether during the day to reap the benefits of fasting. But again, if you're new to fasting, a few small snacks is perfectly okay!

It's Your Choice

Fasting is widely considered among the easier "diets" to follow because it's relatively self-explanatory. However, that doesn't mean it's easy. Choosing a fasting method can be a little complicated.

You might dive into the warrior diet right off the bat, only to find yourself struggling the following day. Take it slow and steady. If you immediately forego sustenance for long periods, you're more likely to falter in your resolve. I've said it before, but it's worth reiterating: Consult a professional before starting an advanced fasting practice.

The key is consistency. No diet is effective if you don't stick to it. Luckily, you have options. Most people find one of the aforementioned plans works for them. You might need to modify or reevaluate your diet plan down the road. That's okay.

Listen to your body. If it's telling you that your plan is too much, give it a breather.

Potential Side-Effects: Why They Happen & What to Do

Some beginning fasters experience cravings, lightheadedness, digestive issues, irritability, frustration, sleep disturbances, bad breath, and mild dehydration.

Luckily, you don't have to. I'll cover some misconceptions in the later chapters. For now, let's discuss why some of these side effects occur.

Cravings

It seems this one might be a given: You're eating much less than you normally would. If it were easy, everyone would do it.

There's a silver lining. One study looked at "1,422 people who participated in fasting practices lasting 4–21 days. They tended to experience hunger symptoms only during the first few days of the regimens" (Kubalan, 2021).

It seems your cravings subside once you get into the fasting habit. Don't worry just yet.

Lightheadedness

Some beginner intermittent fasters report feeling a bit lightheaded when they begin a fasting practice. Again, it's to be expected. You're eating less than you normally would and your body isn't used to the fat-burning process yet.

As your body gets used to your new routine, lightheadedness should subside. Drink plenty of water, tea, and sugar-free fluids throughout your fasting period to mitigate any potential side effects.

Pay attention to how you're feeling and lay down if you need to.

Digestive Issues

Again, your body isn't used to prolonged periods of not eating. Your digestive system was thrown a bit of a curveball. Most of us have eaten three meals a day for most of our lives, so it makes sense that your body needs a little recovery time.

You might experience infrequent bowel movements or slight stomach pain. Fasters report that fiber-rich foods and gut-healthy supplements help with digestive side effects.

As I often say: Pay attention to your body. If you experience serious changes in your digestive routine, see a medical professional.

Irritability & Frustration

You might feel more "short" than normal. Don't snap at your neighbor over their unmowed lawn quite yet; irritability is a short-term side effect of intermittent fasting.

Periods of calorie restriction may lead to anxiety and irritability, though these feelings subside over a short period of time.

A study of 52 women found that most were more irritable during an 18-hour fast. But, following the fast, the women "experienced a higher sense of achievement, pride, and self-control at the end of the fasting period than they reported at the start of fasting" (Kubala, 2021).

Sleep Disturbances

Few people report sleep disturbances while fasting, but it's something to be aware of. It affects people differently.

A recent study showed that 15% of the 1,422 participants who participated in an intermittent fasting habit experienced certain changes in sleep. Some participants woke up at odd intervals while others couldn't fall asleep as they normally would.

The same study shows that sleep disturbances subside within the first few weeks of a fasting routing; keep at it!

Additionally, other studies show the opposite results. It seems disturbances in sleep affect everyone differently.

Pay attention to your body.

Bad Breath

When our bodies enter fat-burning mode, our bodies produce acetone as a byproduct, which makes our breath smell a bit funky. You might notice an odd metallic taste and some report breath smelling a little like nail polish remover.

It's an unfortunate reality, but a breath mint or a cup of spearmint tea should quell your worries.

Mild Dehydration

Our bodies go through autophagy during a fast, which can lead to increased water output. Not only that, but we're consuming fewer water-containing foods.

When we don't properly hydrate and make up for possible electrolyte imbalances, our bodies cannot function as they normally would.

If you're experiencing bad breath, headaches, poor concentration, odd or unusual cravings, poor mood, fatigue or lethargy, or dry, chapped lips, reach for some water.

Hydrate during a fast. Electrolyte imbalances are likely causing many of the aforementioned side effects.

You can't drink enough fluids!

Your Fasting Journey: Revamp Your Mindset

As I said, fasting isn't starvation, nor is it meant to be restrictive. Many people rely on fasting to maintain a healthy weight and mindset, and so can you.

Fasting is a sort of blanket diet; other popular diets are more restrictive in terms of what you can and cannot eat. Fasting is different–you choose how you eat, when you eat, and what you eat. It's the timing that's truly important.

Fasting changes your body in many ways: Your metabolism shifts, cravings vary, and your fat distribution changes (for the better!).

It does come with a few side effects and disclaimers, but there are many ways to combat these. Pay attention to what's happening in your body. If you're feeling too hungry, have a small snack. It's okay to "break" a fast if you're overwhelmed. Try to stick to it as much as possible. Consult your doctor if you're in over your head.

Chapter 2:
Changing Your Mind

"Do something every day that is loving toward your body and gives you
the opportunity to enjoy the sensations of your body."

— **Golda Poretsky**

What you eat fuels your body. Your body, once well-fueled, sends signals to your brain. These signals may be good or bad depending on what we eat, but we'll go into more detail later.

Our brain holds our thoughts, feelings, and rationalizations. If we're not paying close attention to our bodies, our thoughts and emotions take a hit.

Scrap the notions you carry about intermittent fasting; it's not simply a weight loss or wellness tactic. It's a powerful way to connect with yourself.

Fasting, when approached properly, is a means of cleansing. Our bodies take a lot of heat.

As we get older, our laundry list only grows. We juggle family, friends, work, chores, etc. I could go on, but you get the gist. And, as we reach our late 40s, menopause throws a pretty big wrench in that laundry list.

In a brief interview, Linda H., an avid menopause-age intermittent faster told me that, "I began intermittent fasting to lose some weight, but I had no idea how cleansed and fresh I'd feel. I felt horrible waking up and I had so much negativity. I'd snap at my husband, and I felt helpless. It's not a cure, but I highly recommend it to anyone."

Life throws roadblocks in our path. Continuous setbacks lead to self-doubt and negative energy.

Dispelling that negativity is up to us.

In this chapter, I'll discuss just a few of the many holistic, spiritual, and health benefits that accompany proper fasting habits. I won't stop there; this chapter covers what to expect, when to start, and, more importantly, how to cope.

Some of us are skeptical of holistic and homeopathic practices, and that's alright. We can't know how something will benefit us until we try it.

You're in control of your thoughts and feelings. It's time to change your mindset.

Is It Time to Cleanse?

Yes.

I'm not talking about the celebrity Master Cleanse popular in the mid-2000s; I'm talking about the comprehensive benefits of healthy cleansing.

Cleansing isn't a fad diet. It's a lifestyle.

We're all looking for a quick fix. We want immediacy and quick results. Unfortunately, that's not the way our bodies work. Disregard the billboards and Maxicut ads. Focus on steps you can take to make yourself a better you.

Nevertheless, many are interested in the weight loss benefits of cleanses. And yes, you'll likely lose weight throughout the process. Any practice involving restriction or dietary changes triggers weight fluctuations, but those changes reverse when we quit the diet.

That's where cleansing and fasting come into play. As I said, cleanses are a practice. Following a cleanse, and more importantly, understanding what to expect, is the key.

Before we dive into body changes and benefits, let's explore how, when, and what you need to know to get started.

The Physical: Is Your Body Telling You to Cleanse?

Do you feel lethargic, bloated, groggy, or heavy? Now, when I say heavy, I'm not referring to your weight.

Do your arms feel cumbersome? Do your legs feel stiff while you walk?

It's time for a cleanse.

Is exercise arduous? Are you struggling to get out of bed in the morning?

It's time for a cleanse. You're not alone.

Are you in the midst of menopause?

It's time for a cleanse.

Life throws things our way: Bills need to be paid, errands pile up, the food needs cooking, you get the gist. It's a lot, and all of life's intricacies and anxieties don't seem to evaporate when we reach a certain age (or any age, for that matter).

Life's stressors don't just negatively affect our brains and minds, they affect our bodies.

Within your body are two types of toxins: endotoxins and exotoxins. Endotoxins are internal molecules made by your body. They're byproducts of your normal mechanisms. However, exotoxins are a little less innocuous. Exotoxins come from outside the body; they're derived from the air we breathe, the foods we eat, and the environments we occupy.

We ingest, absorb, and consume toxins all day, and a cleanse is how we get rid of them.

Fasting comes with a myriad of benefits, and we've covered those in detail in chapter one. Fasting is great for those struggling with mood, concentration, high blood pressure, insulin sensitivity, high cholesterol, headaches, and chronic diseases.

These aren't the only signs you need a bodily cleanse. Let's look further.

Are you experiencing bloating after eating, diarrhea, or sugar cravings?

Are you experiencing belly weight gain, headaches, water retention in your legs and feet, severe seasonal allergies, inappropriate sweating, or muscle aches?

Are you experiencing acne, dry skin, rashes, itchiness, or large dark circles under your eyes?

If you're anything like me, you answered yes to one, if not many more of these common fasting detox signs.

It's time.

Keep in mind that fasting and cleansing may make exercise more difficult. Maintaining a healthy exercise routine, even one as simple as going for a few weekly walks, is an important part of any healthy diet or lifestyle.

When we fast and cleanse, we consume fewer calories than we would otherwise. Calories are units of energy that fuel our bodies. Exercise burns calories, so when we consume fewer, our muscles have less to work with.

With new cleanses and dietary changes come fluctuations in nutrient levels. It's nothing to be concerned about, but it is something to keep in mind.

For example, many beginner cleansers might experience changes in electrolyte levels. Electrolytes like calcium and sodium are responsible for aiding certain body processes, including cognitive function.

Always check with a medical professional before beginning any diet, cleanse, or nutritional routine. Ensure you're consuming adequate carbohydrates, protein, and fat to maintain your bodily processes.

You come first.

The Brain: Is It Telling You It's Time?

Cleanses go far beyond the physical; we must mentally prepare for cleansing.

Menopause is mentally draining. Your body is changing, and sometimes these changes become overwhelming. You might experience negative thoughts, self-doubt, and anguish.

Do you struggle with gratitude? Do you feel uncomfortable or guilty? Do you feel angry when communicating with others?

If so, that's your negativity talking. It's time to cleanse.

If you feel you're becoming a more negative person, a cleanse is a great way to release negative energy. We don't want to be "glass-half-empty people." Pessimism doesn't benefit us.

Negativity begins with our brains. Think about this. You wake up in the morning and place your feet on the floor. It feels cold and you frown. You roll your eyes and get up, albeit begrudgingly. You feel agitated and anxious.

You meander to the kitchen and begin brewing a pot of coffee. You open the container, about to scoop the grounds into the filter, but the container is nearly empty. You toss it in the trash and roll your eyes once more.

While getting dressed, you find yourself at odds with your body. Your pants might not fit like they used to or perhaps your skin is a little less clear than it was a few years ago.

You're irritated. You're angry. You're bitter.

You've woken up and accepted negativity and, as a result, that negativity clouds your thinking for the remainder of your day. That's no way to live.

If you relate to this image, it's time to change your life.

When we "thrive off of negativity, drama and conflict, it's a clear sign [we] need a spiritual detox" (Fosu, 2022). Your energy may be trapped in an unconscious, yet dangerously negative cycle.

Luckily, you control how you get out of it.

An influx of negative thoughts isn't the only sign your body is ready for a detox; if you're struggling to control what you say, it's time.

Actions might speak louder than words, but words carry a great deal of weight. Our language reflects our reality. If we feel upset, it's reflected in our inflection. If you're sad, others take notice.

A healthy spirit "thinks before it speaks" (Fasu, 2022). You care about others, and that's an admirable quality, but we need to check and filter our language before we can maintain and build healthy relationships.

We need a filter. That's simply reality. Think about what the world would look like if no one had a verbal filter.

Let's say you pitch a new marketing idea to your supervisor. You know it needs a bit of work (it might be under researched, etc.), but you note that in your pitch. Regardless, you're pretty excited about it.

"That's the dumbest idea I've ever heard," they reply. You feel horrible. Anyone would.

We need a filter to function and maintain decorum. That's simply life.

If you feel you're struggling to think before you speak, it might be time for a cleanse. I'll further discuss the cognitive benefits of cleansing later but remember, it's all related.

You might struggle with motivation, and that's another sign. I'll admit that motivation is complex.

And of course, we can't be motivated all the time. Most people struggle to remain motivated throughout the week. You might wake up one Saturday and opt for a "lazy day," which is perfectly acceptable.

But we can't rely on caffeine and deadlines to keep us motivated. It comes from within.

Motivation is a powerful way to control your life.

The Spiritual: Are You in Touch With Yourself?

You might be thinking, "Yes, obviously," but that answer in itself is a sign you need to check in with your spirit.

I'm not referring to your religious beliefs, though if you feel connected with a certain belief system and find yourself struggling, it's time to check in and detox.

The word spiritual has nothing to do with religion, at least, not in the traditional sense. Spirituality refers to how you relate to your soul and your being; it refers to your thoughts and feelings about the world around you.

Do you notice others walking along the street, or do you keep your eyes focused on your path? Do you feel a connection with others? Do you notice yourself detaching from your thoughts and feelings? Do you feel your habits aren't serving or bettering your life?

If you answered yes to any of these questions, it's time to cleanse.

Sleep is another indicator of our spiritual health. It might seem counterintuitive, but our sleep patterns indicate a state of rest and well-being. Many women report that, during menopause, their sleep patterns fluctuate. They can't fall asleep, or when they do, they can't stay asleep.

When you fall asleep easily, it's a sign your mind is at rest. You're at ease with your life and your beliefs. You can probably remember a few (or many) times you couldn't fall asleep. Your thoughts raced right past your conscious mind; you couldn't control them. Maybe you were concerned about a family member or a large project at work. It didn't feel good.

During menopause, the hormones in your brain change. Our cycles fluctuate and rest and relaxation seem to be a distant memory.

If you're struggling with sleepless nights or days you can't seem to peel yourself out of bed, try cleansing.

Cleansing itself began as a spiritual practice. Civilizations have relied on cleaning and fasting for centuries as a means of reconnecting with oneself.

It's been around much longer than the Master Cleanse, I can tell you that.

Don't Overdo It

"Everything in moderation" is a familiar phrase to us all. There's truth to it.

Fasting is a habit, and habits are best incorporated slowly. If you suddenly gave up caffeine cold turkey, you're more likely to reach for the coffee pot after just a few short days.

Start slowly. Begin reducing the amount of sugar you eat. When we lower our sugar intake, our bodies begin to produce ketones, which help ease us into a fasting routine.

I'll admit that the Keto flu is no joke. It's relatively normal to feel lethargic, cranky, and a little out of it. That's why we take it slow. Baby steps lead to big strides and small habits pave the way for larger ones.

Begin adjusting the time you start eating in the morning. If you normally eat a breakfast sandwich at 7 AM, try aiming for 7:30 or 8. If work gets in the way, pack your breakfast and take it with you.

Increase the interval by thirty minutes each week. You might find the switch between 8 AM to 8:30 is a breeze, but your transition to 9 AM or 10 is a little more difficult. Pay attention to your body and what it's telling you, thirty minutes at a time.

Drink plenty of fluids. Now I don't mean smoothies or Starbucks drinks; start with water or tea. Fluids help balance your electrolyte levels, which, in turn, minimizes the fatigue and anguish you feel when getting started with fasting or cleansing.

Your body needs time to get used to fasting the same way you needed to get used to waking up for work.

I'll cover some ways to combat side effects later in the book. Get yourself thinking about how you can start.

Trust the process.

So Why Cleanse? What Do I Get Out Of It?

I've discovered some signs it's time to try cleansing and fasting, but what are the benefits? Together, we discussed some links between menopause and fasting in the last chapter, but it's time to take it a step further.

Listen to your body. You're more than your weight. It's time to take charge.

Fasting & Cleansing the Brain

Thousands of years ago, humans couldn't simply get into their cars and head over to the grocery store. For millennia, we hunted and gathered our food.

Now, grocery stores and restaurants are readily available, but our bodies haven't adjusted to our culture.

Let's check it out.

Fasting & Brain Cells

Our brains benefit from fasting on an evolutionary level. We had to survive without a constant supply of food, and, more importantly, we had to stay alert. You might initially feel lethargic after a few hours of not eating, but over time, our brains become accustomed to a fasting state. You become more efficient.

While fasting, our bodies transition from using carbohydrates in the form of glucose to fuel our bodily mechanisms to using ketones, which are "a type of acid produced by the liver from fat" (Putka, n.d.).

You might've heard of the Keto diet, which works the same way but isn't quite as sustainable as an intermittent fasting cleanse.

Studies show those who begin fasting experience an increase in certain protein markers that indicate increased production of what some call "baby brain cells."

While human studies regarding the increased production of baby brain cells are limited, researchers study those fasting during Ramadan as an alternative. Many participants in observational studies experienced increased memory, functioning, and learning skills, suggesting an increase in brain cell production (Gudden et al., 2021).

Science doesn't lie. Long periods of fasting trigger brain cell production and stimulation.

It's quite literally science.

Cognition and Mood

It doesn't stop there. Fasting and cleansing may improve mental clarity and mood.

Again, it's evolutionary. When we were responsible for finding food, our brains needed to remain sharp at all times. After long periods of fasting, our ancestors needed food and, more importantly, they needed the brainpower to find it.

That's why we feel clearer during a fast.

Women in the throes of menopause who fast for extended periods report feeling more awake, alert, and motivated.

Mental Disease and Decline

No one enjoys getting older, nor do we enjoy feeling sick. Luckily, intermittent fasting is here to help.

There's evidence suggesting that fasting can improve or control seizures in those suffering from epilepsy.

But it's not just epilepsy; intermittent fasting plays a role in preventing the onset of mentally degenerative diseases like Alzheimer's, Dementia, and Huntington's Disease.

One study looked at fourteen participants suffering from mild signs of cognitive decline. The participants were injected with a ketone derivative after a mild fast and underwent neurological tests to gauge the results.

The participants showed an increase in performance on these tests. In another study, researchers found that a three-year prolonged fasting "diet enhanced cognitive functioning in older adults with mild cognitive impairment compared to age-matched adults who irregularly practice [prolonged fasting] and age-matched adults who do not practice [prolonged fasting]" (Gudden et al., 2021)

While fasting, nerve cells in our brains enter resource conservation mode. When we eat, they rapidly regenerate, and neuron function increases. Fasting puts this process to work, and in our brain's favor.

Fasting and Mental Health

Our mental health fluctuates throughout our lives, especially when our bodies are going through changes. Menopause triggers chemical changes in the brain, and these changes negatively affect our mental health.

Don't panic just yet– fasting is a great way to improve your mental health.

While we fast, our bodies hold onto fewer "toxic materials [that flow] through the blood and lymphatic system, improving our cognitive abilities" (Brennan, 2021). All of the energy we normally allocate toward food digestion is used by our brains, providing clarity.

Brain fog and confusion are uncomfortable and frustrating. Fasting helps you gain a more positive perspective.

I discussed fasting's role in our spiritual well-being in the last section, but it's time to look further. Fasting helps your body get rid of diseased, tired cells, paving the way for new cell growth.

Some experts believe that fasting redistributes nutrients and powerful electrolytes in the body; we hold onto "precious vitamins and minerals while processing and getting rid of old tissue, toxins, or undesirable materials" (Brennan, 2021).

Last, but certainly not least, fasting improves willpower. Diets and lifestyle changes are difficult; it takes a while to form a habit. But more than that: They're complicated choices. We choose how we act, how we feel, and what we do daily.

On a basic level, fasting changes the way we see ourselves. I'm not talking about who you see in the mirror, I'm talking about your productivity and mindset. When we make positive conscious choices, we feel better about ourselves, and, in turn, our willpower improves.

When you have a particularly productive day at work, you feel pretty good, right?

Fasting, Cleansing, and Metabolism: The Be-All Breakdown

Fasting is most commonly associated with weight loss. I'll admit, that's why I started. I'll start with weight, but remember, you're more than the number on the scale.

Those beginning intermittent fasting report weight loss of between 3 and 8% of their previous body weight in the first 3-6 months. That's a lot.

But it goes a step further. Many diets offer weight loss, but these diets pale in comparison to intermittent fasting. Those practicing intermittent fasting experience a greater loss of fat in their abdominal area, a lower loss of lean body mass, a decrease in bodily inflammation, and an improvement in fasting insulin levels (Williams, 2018).

We often associate our metabolism with weight loss, but it goes far beyond that.

Basal Metabolic Rate, otherwise referred to as BMR, refers to all the processes your body unconsciously undergoes while fasting. We breathe, our blood pumps, our nerves fire, and our muscles rejuvenate. Unconscious bodily processes use the majority of our daily calories.

But your BMR fluctuates throughout your life. BMR increases during puberty, pregnancy, or times of stress. As we enter menopause, it steadily declines.

Unfortunately, many traditional diets lower BMR over time. Intermittent fasting doesn't fall into that category. Intermittent fasting is a cycle, not a life-change overhaul. Because you alternate between periods of normal eating and fasting, our bodies don't "get used" to the diet, making it more effective over time.

Fasting gently increases your BMR. When your BMR increases, your body readily burns fat, metabolic function increases, hormones become more regulated, and sleep quality improves.

Preparing for a Fast

You know by now how cool fasting is, but what should you expect? How do you prepare?

Here are a few things to keep in mind while preparing for and beginning a fast. It's okay to struggle a little. That's why we prepare.

Drink Fluids

Your body might become dehydrated during a fast. We obtain a lot of water from the foods we eat daily; much more than you might think. Drink unsweetened tea, water, black coffee, and other calorie-free beverages to manage your electrolytes and avoid fatigue and headaches.

I'll cover fluids in more depth in the later chapters. For now, focus on drinking plenty of water throughout the day.

Think About How You'll Break Your Fast

It might seem odd to think about this early, but none of the fasting methods I'll discuss last forever.

After a long fasting period, you'll feel a little hungry, tired, and cranky. Don't reach for a huge cheeseburger just yet; break a fast gently. Your body isn't used to solid food and you don't want to overdo it.

Try simple, yet nutritious meals like brown rice and chicken or a nice salad with tofu. Your body needs a little time before you load up on your comfort foods of choice.

Pay Attention & Adjust

Many fasters report an increased ability to check in with their bodies during a fast; you're more in tune with your cravings and how you'll combat them. It's pretty cool.

But it's science. Fasting cleanses your body, and fewer toxic chemicals run through your blood. Resultingly, your brain can access a healthier blood supply, leading to mental clarity and more positive thinking.

It might take a few days or a few fasting periods to reap the full benefits of this change, but as your body gets rid of harmful toxins, "your brain has access to a cleaner bloodstream, resulting in clearer thoughts, better memory, and increased sharpness of your other senses" (Breenan, 2021).

Use this clarity to your advantage. If you're feeling a little hungry around the twenty-hour mark, take notice. Are you hungry because you're just bored? Or are you really, truly hungry?

Some choose to keep a fasting journal to write down their thoughts and feelings during their journey. Whether you choose to do so is up to you, but for many, it's a powerful way to check in with yourself.

Not only that, but studies also show that fasting redistributes your body's nutrient stores. Your cells and tissues hold onto the good stuff, like vital vitamins and minerals, but flush out toxins and diseased tissues. Fasting heals you from the inside out!

Use your new mindset to your advantage. Beginning a fast isn't easy, but the benefits outweigh the costs.

What to Expect Hour by Hour

So, what should you expect to feel during a fast? What really happens? In this section, we'll discuss the fasting process, hour by hour.

Hours One to Four

Our bodies remain relatively stable between hours one through four; it's the same timeframe between lunch and dinner. It might feel pretty normal.

This timeframe is called the anabolic growth phase. Your body is busy using up the energy you just provided for your normal bodily processes.

During hours one through four, your pancreas produces insulin, allowing your body to use the glucose provided by your meal to store energy.

Hours Four Through Fifteen

Here's where it gets interesting. After four hours, your body has used up most of the remaining energy from your last meal and enters catabolic breakdown; the body releases nutrients from storage and uses them as an alternative energy source.

You're not quite in fat-burning mode yet, but you're getting there.

Hour Sixteen: The Final Countdown

Around hour sixteen, your body begins using fat for energy in a process known as ketosis.

Some enter ketosis more quickly than others. If your last meal consisted of Ben and Jerry's Half-Baked ice cream and two slices of chocolate cake, it may take a bit longer to enter fat-burning mode. Don't worry, you'll get there.

Autophagy paves the way for new tissue formation. It's like wiping a cluttered whiteboard; this process reduces your long-term cancer risk and signs of aging.

You might begin to feel lethargic and cranky around this time; again, don't fear! Once your body enters full-blown ketosis (around the 24-hour mark), you'll experience the mental benefits of fasting. You won't notice the elusive "keto flu" anymore.

Hours Sixteen Through Twenty-four

Your body began producing ketones in the last stage and now the process is in full force. Your liver's glucose stores are nearly depleted, and fat-burning spikes.

You'll still feel relatively energized but pay attention to your body. It might not be a great idea to run a half marathon during this timeframe. You don't need to conserve energy necessarily; just be conscious of how you're feeling.

Taking care of yourself comes first.

Hours Twenty-four Through Seventy-two

You'll begin reaping the cognitive benefits of fasting between the first and third day of a prolonged fast.

Certain neurological chemicals improve and support the growth of new neurons, given you maintain the intermittent fasting cycle.

The ketone bodies your body produces become your brain's primary energy source. Our brains like glucose, but, in many ways, ketone bodies do a better job. You'll experience clarity, alertness, and increased motivation.

Of course, contact a medical professional before trying a prolonged fast. The benefits are pretty amazing, but you'll still maintain those benefits if you choose a short-term fasting method.

Listening to Your Body: How to Move Forward

I noted the importance of listening to your body a few times throughout the chapter, but I'm going to bring it home.

Fasting is as much a spiritual practice as it is a dietary one; the practice helps you tune in to how you're feeling, what you're feeling, and why you might be feeling that way.

Think about your motivations: Why do you want to fast? What is your goal?

Settle into a comfy chair or lay on your bed. Get comfortable. I mean *really* comfortable. Dim the lights and perhaps light a candle. Remove any distractions from your space.

Close your eyes and listen to your heartbeat. If you can't quite hear it, that's okay. Focus on the way you're sitting or lying; pay attention to your chest moving up and down with each consecutive breath.

Try conscious breathing and practice mindful breaths. Conscious breathing involves an awareness of what's around you and how your breath affects your mind.

Think about how the chair is supporting you. How do your arms and legs feel? What's going on inside your body?

Some people like to move from their feet up. Think about your toes releasing the tension, followed by your legs and abdomen. Release the negative energy from your chest, arms, and head. Feel what your body is telling you.

When you're ready, take a deep breath and open your eyes. You'll feel clear, calm, resolved, and light. But not only that, the practice of conscious breathing prolongs feelings of clarity throughout the day.

Try this practice before and during your fast. Some like to meditate this way daily, but the frequency is up to you.

Your body connects to your brain which connects to your thoughts, feelings, and emotions. It's all intertwined.

Fasting isn't simply for weight loss (though it's okay if that's your initial intention), it's a spiritual, cleansing practice, and should be treated as such. Focus on the cognitive benefits of fasting; these come before the number on the scale drops.

You have control of both your body and mind.

Chapter 3:
A History of Intermittent Fasting

"Your body is a temple, but only if you treat it as one."

— Astrid Alauda

My journey toward intermittent fasting didn't begin as an intentional one. I had a habit of skipping breakfast and waiting to eat until lunch in my early twenties and thirties.

Those around me thought it was a horrible habit: Breakfast is the most important meal of the day, right?

Not necessarily.

Needless to say, I didn't intend to begin intermittent fasting, nor did I know what it was. I thought I was just saving a bit of time in the mornings.

I began to feel a little different. At least, different than how I felt before skipping breakfast.

My thoughts were clearer. I didn't need three cups of coffee to wake up in the morning (though I certainly love a good cup of joe). I felt energized, alert, and awake.

But not only that, I felt in tune with my body. I understood how I felt to a degree I hadn't while I ate a well-rounded pancake breakfast. When I was anxious, I understood what to do and how to cope. When I felt depressed or distraught, I knew why.

I couldn't understand why I felt that way, but I liked it. And, over time, I learned more about my habit. It was intermittent fasting, and I had no idea.

It's important to note that intermittent fasting isn't the only diet I've tried. I experimented with juice cleanses, restrictions, and low-fat diets.

Like many Americans, I struggle with body image; diet culture plays a role in how I look at myself in the mirror.

Diets have become a sort of "trend" over the past few hundred years. There's nothing trendy about them.

There's nothing stylish about restriction.

Diet Culture: The Weird, the Odd, and the Crazy

Fad diets have been around for a while, but none have withstood the test of time. Some fad diets sound outlandish, while others seem a bit more justified. Remember, your health isn't a trend. Feeling better never *truly* goes out of style.

In the 11th century, William the Conqueror promoted what he called the 'alcohol diet.' For years he lived in excess, so it's no surprise that, near the end of his life, he grew obese. He went on a "liquid diet," and not a healthy one.

He began drinking nothing but alcohol and consumed very few calories from food. You can imagine this didn't go very well. Alcohol is dehydrating, and wine contains few nutrients. He died shortly after beginning the "diet."

Liquid diets are still popular, but they've evolved. In the 20th century, Lord Byron, a prominent poet, promoted the apple cider vinegar diet, which "instructs people to drink a mixture of equal parts honey and vinegar" (Wdowik, 2017). And yes, apple cider vinegar is still a popular diet tactic, but, at that time, it wasn't sustainable.

Beyonce promoted the Master Cleanse diet in the early 21st century. The Master Cleanse diet was similarly extreme; followers consumed "a mixture of lemon or lime juice, maple syrup, water, and cayenne pepper six times a day for at least 10 days" (Wdowik, 2017).

Pretty crazy, right? We're just scraping the surface.

In the 20th century, the tapeworm diet grew in popularity. Dieters would swallow a tapeworm and let it eat the food they'd consumed throughout the day. It was relatively effective, yet absolutely harmful to the person's digestive system.

I shudder at the thought.

Throughout the 20th and 21st centuries, the cotton ball diet's popularity grew and receded. Followers would simply eat cotton balls when hungry. It didn't last long–many cotton ball dieters suffered bowel obstructions and other dangerous complications.

In the 21st century (yes, you heard that correctly), Breatharianism became prominent. Those practicing this "diet" believed that sustenance wasn't necessary, and followers believed that light and air were all they needed to become healthy.

While this diet sounds like an extreme version of intermittent fasting, it's not. Followers wouldn't eat at all, and many suffered from starvation and nutrition-related illnesses.

Diets come in and out of fashion just like jeans or hairstyles; they range from crazy to chaotic, and few are effective long-term.

However, there's one diet that withstands the test of time. You've guessed it: intermittent fasting.

A History of Intermittent Fasting: Stepping Back in Time

We've discussed the difference between intermittent fasting and other dietary practices, but how did it start? Why was it used?

Intermittent Fasting in Ancient Times

Fasting began as a healing ritual. Philosophers like Hippocrates, the father of modern medicine, and philosophers Plato and Aristotle supported fasting.

They believed it to be a "universal instinct to several kinds of illnesses" (Heffernan, 2020). Beyond illness, early proponents of fasting believed it held cognitive benefits, and they were right.

Other supporters of fasting believed in its healing capabilities. Ancient proponents believed fasting prompted "purification, mourning, sacrifice and enhancement of knowledge and powers" (Hameed, 2022).

Fasting is an ancient practice used by prominent world religions, including Islam, Judaism, and Christianity; it dates back thousands of years.

Fasting & Judaism

Fasting in the Jewish faith began thousands of years ago and remains a common practice in modern Jewish tradition.

Those practicing Judaism celebrate Rosh Hashanah, the Jewish New Year, with ten days of repentance; they also observe Yom Kippur, the Day of Atonement.

Yom Kippur is a fasting holiday in the Jewish faith, and "involves grieving for sins committed in the past year as well as praying for forgiveness" (Hameed, 2022). Those observing Yom Kippur fast for 25 hours and abstain from sex, bathing, and drinking for the duration of the fast.

Fasting is a means of connecting with one's sins and personal misconceptions. It's a reflection skill.

Fasting & Christianity

Early Christians fasted during certain holidays and religious periods, the most prominent of which is Lent.

Lent is a Catholic practice that honors Jesus' forty-day fast before his execution. Though few Catholics still follow complete fasting, they abstain from certain foods and drinks during lent to honor their sacrifice.

Those fasting deny themselves certain comforts to strengthen their spirit and honor their bodies. It's not a diet, but a spiritual practice.

Fasting & Hinduism

Those practicing Hinduism believe that the "denial of [one's] physical needs" yields spiritual gains and clarity. Fasting is meant to "[establish] a harmonious relationship between the body and the soul" (Hameed, 2022).

They believe that worldly pleasures and indulgences prevent one from attaining spiritual enlightenment.

Those fasting in Hinduism practice fasting on Ekadasi days, which refer to the "11th day of the lunar fortnight, twice a month" (Hameed, 2022). Fasting is recommended for those between the ages of eight and eighty; those who cannot fast for health reasons can follow a looser model.

Those practicing Hinduism observe Ekadasi to "destroy all sins and purify the mind." Fasting is "not only as a part of worship; it is also a training of the mind and the body to endure all hardships and to persevere under difficulties and not give up" (Hameed, 2022).

Fasting & Islam

Those practicing Islam [abandon] food, drink, and sexual intercourse from sunset to sundown to honor Allah and gain a connection with their inner being (Hameed, 2022).

Ramadan, the lunar month, is an obligatory practice for Islamic adults. Those observing Ramadan give up temptation and fast. It's customary to fast during the day until sunset.

The practice goes beyond food; those observing Ramadan abstain from lying, harsh language, and sexual intercourse during the day.

Fasting & Buddhism

Fasting is a practice in the Buddhist faith. The Shakyamuni Buddha observed periods of extreme fasting and reportedly ate "only one grain of rice per day" to reach spiritual enlightenment (Visioli et al., 2022).

This practice led to emaciation, and eventually, "Buddha criticized the fasting practiced by Indian ascetics of his day" (Visioli et al., 2022).

In modern times, Buddhist monks do not consume food after noon to gain spiritual well-being and enlightenment.

Fasting in Recent Times

We've established the roots of fasting, but how has it affected us more recently?

In the 19th century, E. H. Dewey claimed that dietary imbalances caused many of mankind's illnesses and tribulations. In this era, proponents of fasting included prominent philosophers who fasted for thirty days or longer.

Prolonged fasts are no longer recommended, but it was believed they reaped health and wellness benefits.

Issac Jennings proclaimed that fasting was more effective than medicine, believing it to be a practice of "hygienic treatment" for the soul. He preached the early methods of fasting, emphasizing the value of a "vegetarian diet, pure water, sunshine, clean air, exercise, emotional poise, and rest" (Visioli et al., 2022).

Later in the 20th century, researchers noticed fasting's benefit to those suffering from obesity. These researchers saw promising results in animals; animal studies seemed to prolong lifespan. Fasting in short sessions was considered a safe weight loss method.

And they were onto something.

Fasting as Holistic Medicine: Healing Your Body & Soul

Fasting is arguably the oldest "diet" in the book; realistically, it's anything but a diet. Early advocates recognized it as a holistic approach to bodily wellness.

It's also important to note that fasting evolved during a time when civilizations had limited communication with one another. And yet, it seemed to develop similarly in different areas of the world.

It was a widespread practice for a reason.

Nowadays, we treat illness differently. The minute we feel the tinge of discomfort that accompanies a headache, we take Ibuprofen. When we feel a slight sniffle, we take Dayquil. When we feel tired, we reach for our Keurig.

Instead of paying attention and working through the feeling, we seek an instant solution. And yes, over-the-counter medications provide immediate relief, but this ideology is equivalent to placing a band-aid over a bullet hole.

It's not a long-term fix.

It wasn't always this way. For millennia, most human and animal species abstained from food when they felt ill. After the illness and discomfort subsided, these species returned to normal eating habits.

Fasting is a restorative practice. Consider sleeping. Most of us sleep every night, at least for a few hours. Your body regenerates itself while you sleep; muscle tissue rejuvenates, neurological pathways restore, and our brains get some much-needed rest.

We don't eat while we sleep. At least, most of us don't. Sleep in itself is a period of fasting and we don't even realize it.

Sleep fasting, otherwise referred to as nocturnal fasting, is a means of "deep and effective detoxification and for repair and restoration" (Mathrick, n.d.).

Unfortunately, when we fall asleep after eating, our bodies don't reap the benefits of nocturnal fasting. Your body focuses on digestion as opposed to cleansing and refreshing your tissues.

Fasting is natural. It's evolutionary. It's holistic.

Instead of using over-the-counter drugs which can contaminate the body, fasting is a means of natural detoxification and cleansing. If the "channels of the body are not blocked due to undisciplined habits of eating and an immoderate lifestyle, the spiritualizing energy is able to act with its full force" (Mathrick, n.d.).

Those practicing fasting don't only reap the benefits I discussed in the previous chapter; they reap the scope of spiritual benefits provided by the practice. It allows you to connect with your inner self while intensifying your beliefs and willpower.

Those who participate in fasting react more positively to stress. It's an evolutionary adaptation, but it's one to take advantage of. When we detoxify our bodies, we detoxify our minds. We react to stress more positively because we feel focused and complete.

Our Modern Relationship With Food

Many Americans have a complicated relationship with food. I fall into this category.

We eat during times of celebration, times of stress, and times of hardship. I love a well-cooked Thanksgiving turkey as much as the next person, and I used to glean satisfaction from binging on potato chips after an arduous day.

We idolize food. We admire it. We think we absolutely *have* to have it. And yes, we certainly do.

However, many Americans idolize it to a degree that's simply not healthy. Phrases like "cheat days," "junk food," and "I've been bad about my diet" are common, but they perpetuate unhealthy ideas regarding what and how we eat.

Fasting asks the follower to abandon their preconceived beliefs about food. They're asked to be mindful and to check in on how they're feeling. Again, it's not about restriction. It's about detoxification and reconnection.

You're familiar with the phrase, "You are what you eat." But that's simply another misconception. You aren't what you eat. You are what you *feel*.

Back to Basics: Reviving the Practice

Fasting as a religious and medicinal practice has been around for centuries. While we no longer believe in the four humors or bathe in public places, our ancestors weren't wrong.

We can use their findings to our advantage. We discussed the benefits of fasting in previous chapters and we've uncovered some common methods to put the practice into action. In this chapter, we connected the dots, so to speak.

Fasting isn't a fad. It's not like jeans or dresses; clothing styles come and go over time. Viable diets simply don't.

The diet industry is just that, an industry. We're taught to believe in the next big invention or product, but this in itself is a dangerous mindset.

Fasting is a means of reconnecting with one's spiritual well-being and health. We can buy protein powder, Advil, and oat milk products until our wallets are virtually empty, but there's another way to heal your body.

You're more than a collection of quantitative numbers and adjectives. You're a whole person and it's your responsibility to treat your body as such.

Chapter 4:

The Unspoken Secrets of Success

"Being a healthy woman isn't about getting on a scale or measuring your waistline."

- Michelle Obama

I stumbled upon intermittent fasting long before I understood what the term meant. I practiced for years and had but a clue!

I noticed some key changes: I felt more energized, comfortable, and alert. But why? After a while, I began to do a bit of research.

I came across the term "intermittent fasting" and had a sort of "aha" moment. It was right there on my screen. I dove into a more intentional method of intermittent fasting; I began the 16:8 practice we discussed in chapter two.

Did I make mistakes? Yes.

Did I learn a lot? Absolutely.

Would I make those mistakes again? You bet.

I, like many other newbie intermittent fasters, fell into a binging trap. I'd forgo food and focus on calorie-free beverages from 8 pm to noon the next day, but I found myself plateauing. I didn't begin the practice solely for weight loss, but it was certainly a secondary consideration.

The number on the scale wouldn't budge, regardless of what I tried or how much I exercised. I wanted to know why.

I was binging. At noon on the dot, I ran to the store across the street and bought a meatball sub and a chocolate chip cookie (which is undeniably the best kind). I ate it with glee before doing a bit more work. At 3 pm I drank a large soda and snacked on some chips from a vending machine. Later, I'd eat my favorite dinner: Steak and potatoes, with a side of corn. I'd finish my non-fasting period with ice cream.

I mistakenly believed that my fast "canceled out" my meals for the rest of the day. I was wrong.

Other fasters report similar issues. I spoke to Diane T, who told me, "I started fasting blind. I understood the fasting part, don't get me wrong. I knew when I should eat and when I shouldn't, but I think I got a little confused. I started with a pretty simple 16:8 plan, and I thought I was doing everything right. I didn't eat anything until noon or even 1 pm. I couldn't lose weight and I still felt a little foggy. I think I was eating the wrong things. I'm a big steak person and love rich foods. I still eat steak sometimes. Well, more than sometimes, but I've learned how to incorporate everything into my fast."

Binging is one of the most common mistakes people make when beginning a fasting routine, but it's certainly not the only one.

We've covered the basics, the ins and outs, and the 'how-to starts,' but we haven't covered the special intermittent fasting secret sauce.

Fasting isn't a complicated concept; for many, it's easy to understand. But, like many other things in your life, adapting intermittent fasting and incorporating it into your routine is much easier said than done.

So how do you go about it? What should you eat after a fast? What are some common misconceptions?

Let's talk about it.

Common Mistakes & Misconceptions

Here's where fasting gets a bit tricky. As I said, there isn't an intermittent fasting 'hack;' there are certainly some tips and tricks, but there's no blanket way to prevent certain side effects.

Listen to your body. Understand the process. Take it slowly.

Here are a few newbie faster mistakes and how you can avoid them!

You Don't Ease Into It

It takes 28 days to form a habit, and oftentimes even longer to break one.

You've been eating a certain number of meals for years. It's called learned hunger; over time, we develop certain eating habits based on learned cues. When you were in your teens and twenties, you learned when to eat and developed your lifelong eating habits.

These habits follow us into adulthood. For me, I get hungry around 3 pm. I don't quite know why, but I have for years. Because of this, I tend to eat dinner pretty late.

If your family regularly ate dinner at 5 pm, you likely hold onto this habit into adulthood. If your favorite food is sushi, it's likely been your favorite for a while.

Habits are difficult to modify. That's why diets are tough. 90% of traditional diets fail; most people don't last six months. In most cases, it's much shorter than that.

Easing into a diet is important. We can't snap our fingers and expect our lives to change.

Luckily, intermittent fasting isn't a diet in the traditional sense. It's a lifestyle. It would be unreasonable (and unsustainable) to dive into a 72-hour fast right off the bat. You might make it for the first 24 hours, but after that, you might falter.

Begin skipping meals. Try increasing your fasting hours by thirty minutes at a time.

Don't dive in all the way just yet. When you've mastered meal-skipping, try a 16:8 model. When you have that down, try the 18:6 or 5:2 method. Review Chapter Two if you need a refresher.

Rome wasn't built in a day. Start nice and slow and low.

You're Consuming Too Many Calories

I made this common rookie mistake during my fasting journey. It's undeniably tempting to break a fast with a McDonald's run or a slice of chocolate cake. And yes, those foods are okay in moderation.

Healthy eating is balanced eating. That's the beauty of intermittent fasting.

Unfortunately, binging is another common reality for newbie intermittent fasters, especially toward the beginning of their journey. After a long 18:6 fast, it's tempting to dive into a large plate of pasta.

We justify it. It's similar to the "cheat day" concept. Fasting periods don't "cancel" what you eat during normal, non-fasting periods. Fasting periods don't change or subvert what you eat normally. Breaking a fast isn't easy. At least, it's not meant to be.

Break a fast with mindfulness. Don't clean your plate just because the food is right in front of you. It takes between fifteen and twenty minutes for your body to register satiety.

Fasting changes the way your body metabolizes food; many intermediate fasters report fewer hunger pangs and discomfort after fasting for a while.

Use your new and improved metabolism to check in with your food intake.

You're Sabotaging With Soda

I'm not saying you can't indulge in the occasional Diet Coke or Sprite, but it's important to understand the effect soft drinks have on your body.

Soft drinks get a bad reputation, and for good reason. You've heard the phrase, "empty calories," and that's a relatively accurate statement. I won't shame you for drinking soda (I do it too), but soda can negatively affect your fast.

Do you feel satisfied after drinking a soda? Do you feel full? Most people don't; here's why. The carbonation in traditional soda "can mask your sense of hunger, which can set you up for being too hungry at your next meal and lead you to overeat" (Coppa, 2020).

Sugar-sweetened beverages raise your sugar tolerance; if you're used to sweet beverages, your taste buds aren't as sensitive to other sweet items, like cookies or cake. After drinking a large coke, you might notice your dessert doesn't taste as sweet.

Drinking soda during a fast isn't advisable; soda completely subverts the benefits of a prolonged fast. It might be tempting to reach for the Diet Pepsi during a 5:2 or warrior fast, but it will undo the work you've put in.

Instead, try to limit your sugar-sweetened beverages to a minimum. Don't drink carbonated drinks during a fasting period. If you absolutely have to have a Coke, save it for your normal eating period. And, even then, try to limit the soda to one 12-ounce glass.

You Aren't Drinking Enough

So you can't drink soda. What are you *supposed* to drink? You have options.

Here's a little secret: food contains water. Most vegetables and fruits are primarily made up of water, and, while we fast, we forego these forms of hydration.

Your body is 70% water, so drink some! Recommended water intake varies from person to person depending on your age, height, weight, and activity level. But, in general, "you should be drinking 2 liters (that's 1/2 gallon) of water per day" (Coppa, 2020).

Water balances your electrolyte levels and supports bodily functions. It's a solvent that aids digestion, excretion, and blood flow.

When we're hydrated, we feel less hungry. Oftentimes hunger cravings mask hydration cravings; in short, you might think you're hungry, but you're really just thirsty.

But again, pay attention to your body. Notice how often you urinate and note the color. Your pee doesn't have to be clear. Shoot for a pale yellow.

You're Not Eating the Right "Fast-Breaking" Foods

Avoid my mistakes. Breaking a fast with a plate full of sausage pizza and brownies is tempting, but it negates the effects of your fast.

Ease back into normal eating. Let's say you're trying the 16:8 method. You've reached the noon mark and it's time to break your fast! You're excited and you run to the vending machine or kitchen and pick out your fast-breaking food of choice. You grab a chocolate bar and dive right in.

You eat it quickly, barely stopping to savor the moment. After a few minutes, you feel sluggish, anxious, and a little bloated.

Your body was in ketosis, and breaking ketosis is uncomfortable. Some people report headaches and digestive discomfort.

When your body is fasting, it becomes a little confused and stops "producing a high volume of digestive juices," so, when you begin eating after a fast, your body needs a little extra time to properly digest what you've eaten (Eckelkamp, 2020).

Some fasters report stomach discomfort, diarrhea, and overall GI upset when breaking a fast.

This brings us to the importance of small, digestible portions. It's tempting to dive right into the chocolate cake you've been craving, but it's important to start small.

Experts recommend that fasters begin breaking their fast with a small healthy snack or soup before eating a full meal.

So, for example, if you're practicing the 16:8 regimen, you would fast until noon and fill up on a nice, healthy, low-sodium, and low-carb soup before eating a gluten-free chicken pasta dinner.

Again, reaching for the cake or cookies is pretty tempting, but this is a common mistake.

Instead of breaking a fast with hyper-palatable foods, consume lean meats, low-fat dairy products, and fruits and vegetables. Eat plenty of protein; protein helps you feel full and maintains your lean muscle mass.

The "fiber from fruits, vegetables, whole grains, and legumes will slow the digestion and absorption of the carbs you eat, so you stay full and energized longer between meals" (Coppa, 2020).

Your body's nutrient stores are running on empty. Use food to replenish these nutrients.

Your Approach Was Too Extreme

I've touched on this before, but it's worth reiterating. Don't go all in immediately. Your body isn't used to fasting, especially if you've never tried it.

Think of it as a friendship. Let's say you meet a new friend through Facebook or a community organization. You chat about the weather, your common interests, and your careers. You wouldn't dive into all of life's intricacies the first time you meet someone. That might be off-putting and a little odd.

Trying an extreme diet is tempting. You've read testimonials and want immediate results. You're not alone! And yes, consuming fewer than 1,000 calories a day will cause weight loss, but it won't be the good kind.

Extreme restriction causes bone loss, especially in women. You want to stay strong and healthy.

Stick with the process. Ease into it.

You're Going Through Caffeine Withdrawals

Have you ever tried to quit caffeine? I certainly have. When I was a bit younger, I noticed my coffee intake slowly increasing. One cup a day led to two and two became three. I barely realized it, but I was a caffeine addict.

Caffeine isn't inherently bad. Some people can quit caffeine with ease, but they're an anomaly. And, if you're a coffee addict like myself, it's hard to quit cold turkey.

So don't.

Caffeine alone won't break a fast, but a mocha chocolate cookie extreme frappuccino with two shots of espresso certainly will. There's nothing in the literature that says you can't drink black coffee or caffeinated tea while fasting.

I recommend it.

Beginner fasters experience sluggishness and frustration when beginning their fasting journey, and caffeine might be the pick-me-up you need to get through a long, 18-hour fast.

Don't overdo it. Cap caffeine consumption to 400 mg a day, or four cups of coffee a day. Four cups is a lot, so try sticking to two or three.

You Work Out Too Hard

Again, it's tempting to go all in when beginning any new diet or lifestyle change. Running to the gym to burn off those calories seems like a great idea, but it can deplete your energy stores in just a few hours.

I'm not saying you should forego exercise altogether. Instead, exercise normally. Your body needs the energy to maintain bodily functions, so don't spend it on an hour-long High-intensity interval training workout.

I'll cover exercise in more depth in Chapter 5. For now, try exercising during your non-fasting period. If you're participating in a 16:8 fasting plan, exercise at 4 pm. Your body needs time to replenish its nutrient stores, so give it a bit of a rest.

You're Overthinking

There's a balance. As a chronically anxious person, I know this firsthand. You don't need to think about every little thing you eat or drink; don't obsess over it. It's easier said than done, and it's tempting to download a calorie-counting app to track everything to the decimal.

Don't fall into this trap.

Many Americans have an unhealthy obsession with food, whether you're a self-proclaimed health nut or not. As a generalization, we think about food quite often. You're focused on your next meal, what you plan to cook for dinner, and what you'll eat this weekend at dinner with your friends.

Food is an obsession. It's an addiction just like any other.

Use mindfulness to overcome this unhealthy mindset. Focus on eating for your body, and not for your own satisfaction. Food is fuel and sustenance. We *need* it to live, but we don't *need* it to feel better about ourselves.

You Give Up Altogether

No lifestyle change is easy. That's a given.

Perhaps you're trying the 5:2 fasting method. It's a little more advanced than some of the others we've discussed, but you've worked your way up and now you're ready.

You've stocked your fridge with the fasting basics: carrots, nuts, apples, chicken breast, etc. You're locked, loaded, and ready to roll.

You do well on the first day. You snack on a few carrots and some hummus and drink green tea until you're sick of it. But, on the second day, you make a mistake. Perhaps a family member brought over some cookies or it's your co-worker's birthday. You look at those cookies and nearly salivate. You need that cookie.

So you eat one. But one becomes two and soon, you've broken your fast. You quit and, for the rest of the day, you eat nothing but cookies, snacks, chips, pretzels, etc. You failed at your fast and you give up altogether.

Check your language. Re-read the previous example. I used words and phrases like "do well," "mistake," "need," "quit," and "failed."

Throw these words in the trash can. They have no space in your fasting vocabulary. The word "failure" has an inherently negative connotation, but there's nothing "failing" about the cookie you ate.

Trade these words for others. Replace the word "mistake" with, "learning experience." Trade the word "failed" for "lapse" or "blunder."

Use language that reflects a positive mindset. Don't beat yourself up. You ate a cookie; you didn't crash your car into the pole on Main Street.

Your fast wasn't a failure because it didn't go as planned. You don't need to give up altogether. Reward yourself for what you were able to do. In this example, you fasted for nearly 30 hours. That's an incredible accomplishment.

Keeping Yourself Full: Food & Drinks

So how do you get through a fast? It's completely possible with a little thought, preparation, and know-how.

If you're a picky eater like myself, you might have some conflicting thoughts about what to eat and drink while fasting. That's okay. You're in luck. The best aspect of intermittent fasting is that you choose what you eat!

This section might be a head-scratcher: Why discuss food and fasting? Isn't fasting the absence of food? Well, yes. You're on the right track. But it's impossible to completely forego nutrients altogether, even if you're practicing Breathenarianism (which isn't recommended).

Don't skip this section just yet; what you eat during and after a fast is nearly as important as the fast itself.

I touched on a few foods and drinks you can consume to maintain and break a fast; here's where we'll dive a little deeper.

Your Fasting Drink Guide

Let's start simple. Drinks are absolutely part of a healthy fasting routine, but again, we have to be conscious of our choices.

Water, Tea, and Coffee: The Starter Pack

Water is a given; we need water to survive. Without it, we become dehydrated, lethargic, and hungry. It seems relatively self-explanatory, but believe me, more people forget to drink water than you'd assume.

Tea is another great beverage; I've discussed it a bit in previous sections, but tea comes with serious benefits. It's worth discussing.

I wasn't a tea drinker until my mid-thirties, but since then, I'm hooked. Tea is a great way to cleanse your body during a fast and to keep you satisfied. Water is great, but sometimes, we need something with a little taste.

Try green, chamomile, earl grey, mint, chocolate, or ginger tea to satisfy food cravings.

I'm not talking about sweet tea; I'm a southern girl myself, but sweet tea will break your fast.

Coffee is great. It's fantastic even. I'd like to personally thank whoever invented coffee. As we discussed, coffee is a part of a healthy fast.

It comes down to science. Coffee can act as an "appetite suppressant and can be used as a meal replacement for breakfast or lunch" (Lett, 2021). Additionally, "coffee consumption can increase ketone production and regulate blood glucose, which enhances metabolic health" (Lett, 2021).

If you're not a coffee drinker, that's okay too. You don't *need* coffee to maintain a fast.

Keep in mind that too much coffee or caffeine can aggravate menopausal hot flashes. Caffeine in high amounts can also cause sleep disturbances, which is another common symptom of menopause. Caffeine dilates your blood vessels, allowing more blood to rush to your head at inconvenient times.

I'm not saying you can't enjoy your morning cup but refrain from drinking coffee throughout the day. Stopping caffeine consumption at 3 pm is a good rule of thumb.

Here's where we mix it up. Bulletproof coffee is a popular choice enjoyed by many following the Keto diet. For those who aren't familiar, bulletproof coffee is drip coffee with a small amount of coconut oil or butter added to prevent hunger pangs.

However, there's a catch. Some believe bulletproof coffee breaks a fast. On the other hand, others believe that, because the calories in bulletproof coffee come from fat, the drink does not raise glucose levels.

Whether or not you indulge in bulletproof coffee is up to you. Choose tasty, fast-friendly drinks.

Apple Cider Vinegar & Bone Broth: Best Kept Secrets

You might be familiar with the apple cider vinegar diet. Some believe a shot of apple cider vinegar (ACV) helps curb hunger cravings. But it's not a diet on its own (and I think it tastes a little odd).

However, ACV is a great addition to a fast. It's nearly calorie-free and "aids digestion, improves insulin sensitivity, lowers blood glucose, and increases satiety" (Lett, 2021).

Don't drink too much ACV; try a small shot when you're feeling particularly hungry.

Bone broth is another popular choice. It's not a soup necessarily, but it's a "rich source of minerals, and will help replenish electrolytes, which are normally lost during a fast. It is also a great source of collagen, which will restore and repair the gut lining" (Lett, 2021).

Some report the protein in bone broth breaks a fast, but other experts feel otherwise. Again, it's up to you to pick a liquid of choice to maintain and prolong your fast.

Salt: The Spice That (May or May Not) Make Everything Nice

I'll explain. Salt seems a little counterintuitive to a fast. And yes, too much sodium can be a real issue. However, there's nothing wrong with a dash of salt.

Electrolyte levels take a bit of a hit during a fast. Luckily, salt is here to help. Salt helps "replenish electrolytes, cleanse the palate and dampen hunger" (Lett, 2021).

However, too much salt can be a real problem: Salt intake is linked to lower bone density in women during menopause.

A sodium intake higher than 2 grams daily has been linked to a 28% higher risk of low bone density in women between the ages of 50 and 60. Lowering your salt intake decreases bloating and brain fog while improving bone density and cardiovascular function.

Don't overdo it. Try a tiny pinch of salt in your beverage of choice to help curb hunger pangs during a difficult fast.

Your Go-to Food Guide

We've discussed a few foods to eat after a fast; let's take it a step further! More information is always better than less.

Before we dive into our mini "Eat this, not that," let's talk about a few things to keep in mind. Again, some of this information might seem a bit repetitive, but again, everyone can use a refresher.

You know by now that fasting isn't a diet so much as it is a lifestyle. But, because it's a lifestyle, it involves some lifestyle changes and thinking alterations.

Begin preparing food at home. Don't groan; eating at home is a fantastic way to control what goes into your food, and, in turn, what goes into your body. Another plus? It's wallet friendly.

Preparing meals at home helps you avoid overly processed foods. Frozen meals and pre-prepared dishes are okay when you're in a pinch, but we can't rely on manufacturers to meet our nutrient needs for us. Cooking is an empowering way to alter your perception of food. It's nourishment, not a reward.

At-home meals don't have to be boring; in fact, I find them pretty fun. When you cook at home, you choose your spices, flavors, and recipes. If you're a fan of red pepper flakes, add them! If you love brown rice (I do), use it in your recipe.

Eat balanced meals. Think back to the food pyramid. Design a meal with a lean protein, a fruit or veggie (both are recommended), a healthy carbohydrate, and fat.

I'll discuss these food groups later in the chapter but keep healthy meal planning in mind.

Eat mindfully. Don't scarf your food down like you're catching a bus. Take time to recognize the food's taste and texture. How do you feel while you're eating? What do you like about the food? What don't you like?

Mindfulness is a powerful practice. Use it throughout your fasting journey.

To Eat or Not to Eat: The Menopause Question

Intermittent fasting is a flexible lifestyle plan, so nothing is entirely "off limits." However, maintaining a relatively healthy diet is always a good idea.

Fasting when combined with proper nutrients can mitigate many potential menopausal symptoms.

Balance is key.

Focus on fruits, vegetables, healthy carbohydrates, and lean proteins. I'll dive into the importance of protein in the next section; right now, let's talk about other components of a healthy diet.

Fruits and veggies are important; you learned this in grade school. What they didn't tell you is how fruits and vegetables relate to fasting and menopause.

In general, fruits and vegetables are full of "vitamins, minerals, phytonutrients (plant nutrients) and fiber" that control your blood sugar, gut health, and lower LDL cholesterol (Castaneda, 2020).

Both fruits and veggies contain prebiotic fiber, so they keep you nice and full throughout the day. Some vegetables, like spinach, kale, and greens contain essential calcium to maintain bone health.

Other vegetables like beans and legumes contain magnesium, folate, and vitamin C to help your body maintain its nutrient stores while fasting. Keeping your body healthy and focusing on positive nutritional habits are fantastic ways to boost your confidence during menopause.

Not only that—fruits and veggies are great fast-breaking foods! Both are low in calories, so they're safe foods for warrior dieters and 5:2 fasters.

Dairy products are also pretty important. Osteoporosis and declining bone density are common causes of menopause, especially as estrogen levels decline. Low-fat dairy products like cheeses and skim milk are great ways to maintain your bone density and can also promote healthier sleep habits! Dairy products are high in glycine, which plays a role in more restful sleep.

Foods like salmon, sardines, and broccoli also contain essential calcium to promote long-term muscular-skeletal health.

Not all carbohydrates are created equal. I don't like the term "bad carbs," but some carb sources are healthier and more beneficial than others.

"Bad carbs" include white bread, fancy pastries, cookies, cakes, and sugary foods. They don't provide the full scope of nutritional benefits available. And yes, it's okay to indulge occasionally, but, in general, focus on more nutritious carbohydrate choices like whole grain pasta or bread, potatoes, fruits, and beans.

Fatty meats like large steaks and processed meats (sausage, etc.) can cause long-term issues related to weight gain and heart disease. Those consuming fatty meats regularly report a higher incidence of hot flashes and headaches. It's okay to chow down on a ribeye once in a while but try to minimize consuming these foods as much as possible.

Spicy foods and hot sauces can worsen menopause symptoms. Your body temperature rises when you eat spicy foods; you're physically hot! Spicy foods can worsen hot flashes, so do your best to refrain from the extra hot sauce on your wings. Use alternative spices like cumin or basil to season meals.

You're well aware that fast food isn't too healthy for you, but consuming large amounts of fast food during menopause can increase your risk of heart disease in just a few short months. If you're busy and can't find the time to cook meals at home, try meal prepping or opting for a salad instead of a Big Mac!

We all love sugar. At least, most people do. I'm a chocolate chip cookie fan myself, and there's nothing wrong with indulging once in a blue moon!

However, some studies point to a link between sugar consumption and frequent hot flashes in women during menopause.

Your body is more likely to develop insulin resistance during menopause, so what might've been a small indulgent snack can become a big problem over time. Higher levels of insulin can cause heart disease and weight gain.

Many menopausal women report more sugar cravings than they did before perimenopause; your hormones are out of whack and your body wants immediate satisfaction.

To conquer cravings, sweeten your foods with honey or maple syrup and try to prepare meals at home. Grab a piece of fruit instead of a candy bar. It's a little difficult–I'll admit it. It's okay to reach for a sugary snack once in a while but try to keep the sugar to a minimum.

Again, these foods aren't inherently bad. Think of various foods as neither black nor white, but as shades of grey.

It's okay to have a little sugary snack following a long fast. Listen to your body.

Menopause, Hot Flashes, and Food: What Gives?

Hot flashes are the most common symptom of menopause, particularly perimenopause and mid-menopause. Hot flashes can be unwelcomed and uncomfortable. Many women report a warming or hot feeling on their face or chest, but others feel it throughout their whole body. Hot flashes can last for up to 10 minutes.

In short, they're not super fun.

Luckily, we have options.

Whole grains, otherwise known as complex carbohydrates, are jam-packed with fiber, riboflavin, and niacin, all of which can help keep you full and keep those hot flashes at bay. Whole grains don't have to be boring—I wasn't an initial fan myself, but whole grain bread, quinoa, and brown rice are delicious when prepared with care.

I'll include some recipes that use whole grains in Chapters 6, 7, and 8.

The Power of Protein

Protein is an important macronutrient, but it often flies under the radar when compared to fat and carbohydrates. Nevertheless, your diet isn't complete without it.

You might be asking, "Why are we discussing protein in particular?"

Protein is an especially important nutrient to intermittent fasters or really any dieter for that matter.

Let's dive right in.

Protein, Satiety, & Cravings

Hunger cravings are an unfortunate reality all fasters are quite familiar with.

Cravings aren't simply a desire to eat, nor are they the feeling you experience when you're hungry (though that's certainly a contributing factor). No. Cravings are your brain's way of telling you it needs a little reward.

However, studies show that protein is a powerful way to curb cravings. One of the best prevention methods is increasing your protein intake.

One study showed "that increasing protein to 25% of calories reduced cravings by 60% and the desire to snack at night by half" (Gunnars, 2019).

Cravings improve your brain's ability to process dopamine, otherwise known as the reward hormone. Protein gives your brain the pick-me-up it needs while healthily curbing food cravings.

Protein makes you feel fuller, especially when compared to its other macronutrient counterparts.

And there's scientific evidence behind this as well. One study noted that when participants increased "protein intake from 15% to 30% of calories [they consumed] 441 fewer calories each day without intentionally restricting" (Gunnars, 2019).

Protein, Muscles, and Bone Health

Satiety isn't the only benefit of increasing your protein intake. Protein is essential for proper muscle development, which, in turn, supports healthy bone maintenance.

Some fasters report losing lean muscle mass while practicing intermittent fasting. Luckily, protein is here to help. Protein helps your body retain the muscle it needs while still losing fat in unwanted places.

Our muscles protect our bones, and scientists believe that those who consume adequate protein maintain bone mass more effectively, preventing osteoporosis.

Protein & Weight Loss

Many people are interested in losing weight; that's not front-page news. Consuming adequate protein boosts your metabolism.

Studies report that those with a high protein intake burn on average 80-100 more calories a day when compared to their low protein eating counterparts. You don't have to think about it.

Studies show that, when all other factors remain the same, overweight participants who increased their protein intake to 30% of their daily calories "lost [on average] 11 pounds in 12 weeks" (Gunnars, 2019).

It's not just about weight loss. Many dieters understand the difficulty of *maintaining* weight loss. You wouldn't want to gain it all back, right?

Another study showed that increasing one's daily calories from protein reduced post-diet weight gain by 50%.

Pretty cool, right?

Beyond Weight Loss: Protein and Body Mechanisms

Let's take it a step further; protein lowers your blood pressure, even when other aspects of your diet remain entirely constant.

Some wrongly assume that protein harms your kidneys. But that assumption is a little outdated. Healthy adults reportedly had no change in kidney function while maintaining a high-protein diet.

However, if you suffer from kidney disease, consult a medical professional before altering your protein intake.

How to Eat More Protein: A Beginner's Guide

Fasting implies a period of restriction, so it might seem a bit silly to discuss what to eat after a fast. However, maintaining a healthy diet and curbing cravings is of interest to any faster, regardless of their chosen fasting method.

Consuming more protein is, again, easier said than done, especially for fasters. We mistakenly believe that fasting is what matters, but what you eat is just as important as what (and when) you don't.

I'll talk about protein and the 16:8 fasting method because it's the most popular. Of course, the same principle applies to any fasting method you choose.

Make the most of your eating window. If you're following the 16:8 plan, choose your meals wisely. Eating two servings of protein, like a piece of salmon or one serving of lean meat, is a great way to replenish your body after a fast.

Your protein intake shouldn't change simply because you're practicing intermittent fasting. It might be tempting to restrict all food groups after a fast, but this is a rookie mistake. Aim for 30% of your daily calories to come from protein, regardless of your chosen fasting.

If you're following a more advanced fasting practice, you might need to get a little creative. Adding protein powder to your drinks or using nuts or tofu to satisfy hunger cravings is a great way to maintain protein intake during a warrior or 5:2 fast.

So how much protein do you *really* need? The general rule is to aim for 7 grams of protein per 20 lbs of body weight. For example, if you weigh 160 lbs, aim for 56 grams of protein a day.

The math is as follows.

160 pounds/20 pounds=8

8 x 7 grams of protein =56 grams of protein

For context, 4 ounces of lean salmon equates to about 33 grams of protein. So, if you have salmon for dinner, you're nearly three-quarters there.

The following foods are examples of animal and plant protein sources. Remember, you can meet your protein goals like a champ!

- Chicken breast
- Nuts, especially almonds
- Greek yogurt
- Low-fat milk
- Low-fat cheese
- Lentils and beans
- Lean red meat (emphasis on the word "lean")
- Protein powders
- Turkey breast
- Shellfish (shrimp, scallops, etc.)

Sleep: The Biggest Secret

Sleep is important. We can't survive without it. You might not need a full eight hours of rest, but the majority of American adults sleep fewer than seven hours a night. That doesn't bode well for the rest of their day.

We talked about the link between sleep and menopause in the earlier chapters; it's pretty important. Many women report changes in their sleep patterns during menopause, especially during mid-menopause.

I spoke to Carrie L., who told us that: "I kept waking up in the middle of the night for no reason. I tried reading a book before bed, eating a good dinner, everything. Nothing really helped. I even tried melatonin and other sleep aids but nothing worked. I didn't get how menopause would change sleep until I was in my early fifties."

You learned the benefits of a great night's rest in grade school, but there's one benefit people forget to mention: weight loss. Those who sleep less than six or seven hours nightly are at an increased risk of a high BMI and weight gain.

Again, it's backed by science.

Sleep affects hunger hormones, causing those who get little rest to feel hungrier; those who receive less than seven hours of nightly sleep are more likely to "consume more calories from high-fat and high-sugar foods (Pullen, 2017).

Conversely, those who receive their beauty rest consume, on average, 385 fewer calories than their restless counterparts. The research suggests that those who receive plenty of sleep feel fuller.

In short, sleep helps moderate your growling appetite, which is especially important during menopause.

It doesn't stop there. Sleep may impact your metabolism, which could be a good thing or a bad thing.

Studies show that lack of sleep may "significantly lower basal fat oxidation in people of different ages, sexes, and body composition" (Pullen, 2017). Those were some big words, but, in short, when you're chronically restless, your body isn't able to burn fat properly, negatively impacting your metabolic rate.

And, on a more practical level, going to bed early helps you avoid late-night snacking. Late-night snacks are delicious; I readily admit it. However, late-night snacking increases your caloric intake.

When you're sleepy, you're more likely to make unconscious choices. You might reach for a bag of dark chocolate chips, but a handful turns into a bagful very quickly.

Here's the kicker: The benefits of sleep become amplified when combined with intermittent fasting. Let's discuss.

Sleep & Intermittent Fasting

Intermittent fasting and sleep go hand-in-hand, though it may not seem that way. Fasting reinforces your circadian rhythms. Our circadian rhythms regulate hunger, appetite, and other bodily functions. It's important.

We discussed human growth hormones in previous chapters; those practicing intermittent fasting have higher levels of HGH, which is produced during sleep.

Human growth hormone "burns fat, restores muscles, and helps the body repair itself at a cellular level," consequently, those practicing fasting wake up after a lovely night's rest feeling energized and refreshed (Leiva, 2019).

Menopause is known to negatively affect one's sleep patterns, and changing human growth hormone levels might be to blame. Hormonal changes during menopause can cause a drop in HGH levels, meaning your body can't rest or reap the benefits of a good night's sleep.

Getting a lovely and restful night's sleep is much easier said than done. We've developed our current sleep patterns throughout our lives. If you identify as a night owl, you've been that way for years.

Intermittent fasting is here to help. Eating a large meal right before bed is tempting, but not recommended. If you begin fasting a few hours before you head to bed, you'll reap more benefits than those who eat later at night. And consequently, a restful night's sleep boosts HGH levels.

It's a cycle.

Pro Tip # 1: Never Go to Bed Hungry

You're likely a little hungry, tired, or cranky after a day of fasting, especially if you're a newbie faster. When we fall asleep hungry, we're focused on food. We want it and we need it.

You've noticed the difference between falling asleep on an empty stomach and falling asleep after a great, healthy meal. The latter is much easier.

Aim to eat your last meal about three hours before heading to bed. Late-night snacking is tempting, but with a little planning, you can overcome your midnight cravings.

Pro Tip # 2: Set the Scene

Sleeping with the lights on or in a loud place isn't easy. If your phone is buzzing, emails are flooding your inbox, and there are sirens outside, you might feel uncomfortable or restless.

Temperature matters too. Our body temperature drops while we sleep; if the temperature in your room is above 70 degrees F, you might find yourself tossing and turning.

Relax before heading to bed. Perhaps take a nice shower or bath.

Studies looking at baths before bedtime show positive results: It boils down to temperature changes. Participants who took a hot bath with a water temperature of around 104 degrees F, tended to fall asleep more readily than their non-bathing counterparts.

If you take a hot or warm bath before going to bed, your body relaxes and becomes more receptive to sleep.

The same studies show that "taking a hot bath or shower before bed could improve certain sleep parameters, such as sleep efficiency and sleep quality," which is especially important for those practicing intermittent fasting and for women during menopause (Semeco, 2020).

Light matters too. Light can influence your body's internal clock, which regulates sleep and wakefulness. If your body is exposed to light on an irregular basis, this can disrupt your "circadian rhythms, making it harder to fall asleep and stay awake (Semeco, 2020).

Light tells your body to stay awake; it's an evolutionary trait. However, the same goes for artificial light: Your phone, Kindle, or nightlight can keep you awake far past your bedtime.

On the flip side, sleeping in the dark tells your body to go to bed. Studies show "that darkness boosts the production of melatonin, an essential hormone for sleep" (Semeco, 2020).

Along that line, eliminate electronics before bedtime, your body will thank you. Electronic devices emit what's called blue light, which can stop or eliminate melatonin production.

Notifications on your computer, phone, or other devices won't help you fall asleep; they'll do the opposite. Constant buzzing, pinging, or blinking can greatly disrupt your sleep/wake cycle, so shut off your phone before turning the lights off.

Long story short, turn off the lights, set your phone to 'do not disturb,' and eliminate distractions. Mitigate any potential noise.

Grab your favorite blanket and cozy up!

Pro Tip # 3: Hydrate

This tip might seem like a head-scratcher; contrary to popular belief, heading to bed dehydrated is linked to lower-quality sleep.

When you're thirsty, your body can't properly relax; it focuses on maintaining hydration, not getting shut eye.

I'm not saying you should hydrate with caffeine. In fact, I'm saying the opposite. Intermittent fasters often rely on caffeine to keep themselves alert and satiated throughout the day, and that's alright! However, drinking coffee, sugary, or soft beverages, or energy drinks can impede your ability to sleep well.

Stop drinking caffeine around 3 or 4 pm. Instead of coffee, try caffeine-free tea. Chamomile tea and other forms of green tea can promote proper rest and relaxation. If you're not a tea drinker, drink plain water or flavored unsweetened water drinks.

Don't drink alcohol before bed either. Alcohol is a stimulant and drinking alcohol before heading to sleep can impede melatonin production.

Here's a disclaimer: Don't drink beverages too close to bedtime. This seems a little counterintuitive, so hear me out—drinking water too close to bedtime can cause you to stay awake. In short, you'll have to run to the bathroom!

Aim to drink tea or water about an hour before your designated bedtime.

Pro-Tip # 4: Consistency

Consistency *is* key.

I'll be the first to admit that I struggle with this one.

Going to bed at erratic times confuses your body. We're creatures of habit after all. It might be nice to sleep in on weekends after a long week of work, family, and errands, but your body isn't used to that schedule.

It's okay to vary a tiny bit: If you normally wake up around 6 am to get ready for the day during the week, aim to wake up before 6:30 am or 7 on weekends. If you normally head to bed around 10 pm, don't stay up until the wee hours of midnight on a Saturday.

Your body likes consistency.

Fall asleep around the same time daily and aim to wake up at the same time. Your body will thank you.

Misconceptions Aside: What Comes Next?

Everything. Once you scrap your preconceived notions regarding intermittent fasting, your body and mind fall into place.

The foods you eat are just as important as the ones you don't. Intermittent fasting is a lifestyle change as much as it is a diet; and, consequently, it should be treated as such.

Mistakes are common; we all make them. Ease into the process and focus on hydration.

Don't reach for the snack cupboard right after a long fast; try opening the refrigerator and grabbing a healthy, protein-rich snack.

It's a balance. Change doesn't happen overnight, nor should we expect it to! It's okay to indulge once in a while. I'm an advanced intermittent faster, but I still love a great chocolate-covered strawberry.

Keep your mindset in check. Notice what you're craving, when you're craving it, and how you feel. There's no sense in beating yourself up. Talk to yourself as you would a dear friend. Treat yourself like the amazing woman you are.

Your body isn't a temple. It operates as a cycle. What we give is what we get.

Give your body the nutrients and rest it needs to be your best intermittent fasting self.

Are you feeling a little more at ease, like someone's in your corner?

Do you feel more comfortable moving through this new life stage?

If you're liking the book so far, please consider helping a fellow

woman and small business owner expand their business! Drop a

review under "Book Review" to help women continue to help women!

Please and Thank You!

Woods Publishing

Chapter 5:

Move More

"Looking after my health today gives me a better hope for tomorrow."

— Anne Wilson Schaef

Exercise is essential. That's not a professionally kept secret. Exercise guidelines vary depending on your weight, activity level, and other environmental factors. However, for most American adults, the Center for Disease Control recommends 2.5 hours of moderate-intensity activity a week.

Here's the catch: Moving doesn't equate to exercise. Moving is the habit of embracing your body and using it to do work for you. On the other hand, exercise is the habit of intentional, scheduled periods you allot to a certain activity.

Weight loss doesn't need to be your motivation for moving more. People move for a variety of reasons, and these may or may not pertain to the number on the scale. However, if weight loss is your motivation to get movin', you're in luck. It's pretty effective.

Additionally, moving can amplify the benefits of intermittent fasting. I'll discuss this more in the chapter, but for now, try answering the following questions.

- How much have you moved today? Why was that?
- Where did you move and why?
- Do you think you could have moved more?
- Do you think you should have moved less?

I've repeated the phrase 'listen to your body' a few times. You might be a little tired of it by now. Regardless of how you feel or whether you're rolling your eyes, *do it*. Moving isn't an option, it's a necessity.

Move more, my friend.

Should I Exercise?

Yes. Absolutely.

We've covered the benefits of intermittent fasting, but you'll find the practice much more effective when you combine it with moving a bit.

The benefits of exercise overlap with many benefits that come from intermittent fasting.

But why? But what? Let's get into it.

Both fasting and exercise lower your blood sugar. When you move while practicing intermittent fasting, you become even less likely to develop insulin resistance when compared to those trying one or the other. In turn, you'll reap more blood-sugar benefits than your sedentary fasting counterparts.

Scientific studies support this ideology: Martin Berkhan, a prominent nutrition professional conducted a study looking at three groups.

The first group, or the C-group, consumed a large, carbohydrate-rich meal right before working out. Their meal was enhanced with important nutrients like Vitamin C and Vitamin D.

The second group, or the F group, practiced what's called fasting exercise; they worked out during a fast. However, after the workout, "they received the same meal as the C group but later on in the day," or a few hours after their exercise (H, 2019).

The third group, otherwise known as the control group, ate the same exact meal, right down to the gram, but didn't work out or fast in any way. The purpose of the control was to test the participant's normal blood sugar levels.

Long story short, the F group, or the fasting group, had improved glucose tolerance and showed lower levels of insulin sensitivity when compared to the two other groups.

The C-group, or the eating and exercise group, saw improvements in these metrics, but not to the degree the F group did in the study.

The control group saw no change in glucose or insulin sensitivity, as expected.

So yes, it works.

If you read the first few chapters carefully, you understand how the human growth hormone works and its (many) benefits. We haven't discussed human growth hormone and exercise; studies show that HGH levels increase after a workout session, leading to a quicker recovery and increased muscle development.

It's like turning the volume up. Your body produces more human growth hormone compared to those who choose not to move during a fast.

Testosterone levels increase when you exercise during a fast. Don't scratch your head just yet; women need testosterone just as much as their male counterparts. Testosterone plays an important role in the development of lean muscle mass.

Unfortunately, any diet can impede your body's ability to maintain lean muscle mass. And yes, intermittent fasting can maintain lean muscle mass more effectively than most diets, but it's still a risk.

It works like this: When your testosterone levels increase after exercise, you'll hold onto essential lean muscle which will, in turn, prevent your body from storing more fat.

Autophagy is one of the most important yet least discussed benefits of intermittent fasting. Some studies show a link between exercise while intermittent fasting and higher rates of autophagy, or cell rejuvenation.

If those facts weren't enough to convince you to get out there, maybe this one will: When combined with intermittent fasting, exercise increases fat burning by about 20% when compared to those practicing one or the other.

Exercise uses glycogen, your body's fuel, to power its movement. So, when you exercise, you burn more fuel, which lessens the time your body needs to enter fat-burning mode.

So, if your motivation is weight loss, you're in luck. Give it a try!

Working Out While Fasting: Disclaimers and Notes

We discussed some disclaimers regarding exercise and intermittent fasting in previous chapters.

Careful mindfulness is important: If you feel your body is telling you to take a break, give yourself some time to ease into it.

Why It May Not Be Effective

Before I talk about how to cope with and mitigate the negative effects of exercising while practicing intermittent fasting, let's talk about a few precautions and disclaimers.

If you've been exercising for a while, you might notice poorer performance while exercising during a fast.

Your body is transitioning from using glucose for energy to using fat, and it needs a little time to get used to the change. If you feel exhausted after your one-mile hike, don't get discouraged. Take it one step at a time.

However, if you've been sedentary for a bit (it's okay, it happens to the best of us), then you might not notice this change.

Some studies show that those practicing intermittent fasting have a more difficult time developing muscle than those who eat 'normally.' However, intermittent fasting did not affect the fasters' ability to maintain existing muscle mass.

Don't be alarmed—this is normal. Many diets have this effect and it's important to note that most existing studies used an exclusively male control group. But again, use caution and take note if you notice anything alarming.

Exercising while fasting may also negatively affect your blood pressure. And, in general, low blood pressure is a good thing. However, when your blood pressure gets a little *too* low, you might become dizzy or lightheaded.

Both exercise and intermittent fasting lower blood pressure, so the combination can cause negative symptoms. If you're feeling as though it's too much, take a break.

How to Do It the Right Way

It's possible; we just have to be conscious.

If you're practicing your first fast (congrats!), avoid high-intensity exercises like running, sprinting, or high-intensity interval training workouts. I'll go into this in more depth later, but for now, focus on trading high-intensity workouts for low-impact ones: walking, slow jogging, and yoga are great places to start.

Weightlifting while fasting is okay, just in short doses. Glucose levels while weightlifting gets a little tricky. When you lift weights while fasting, your muscles won't have access to the glucose they normally would, making the workout a little less effective than it normally would be. Try lifting smaller weights when exercising during a fast.

Focus on your timing. It's not advisable to dive into a brand-new workout routine on your first day of a fasting routine. Try exercises you feel comfortable with; if you love Barre but you're a Pilates newbie, now isn't the time to try a high intensity Pilates class. Don't jump into everything at once.

Along that line, remain flexible with your timing. Planning workouts can be difficult. Perhaps you have to be at work by 7 am, pick up children or grandchildren at 4 pm, make dinner by 6 pm, and get to bed early enough to do it all! There's not always a ton of time, so we have to plan for it.

That being said, if you normally exercise between 4 pm and 5 pm, time your fasting to accommodate that. I briefly discussed fasting during a cardio workout, and I'll go into more detail later in this chapter, but if your goal is to reap the benefits of a fasted cardio workout, try exercising in the morning before you break your fast. If you prefer weightlifting or high-intensity interval training, aim to engage in those activities later in the day after you've broken your fast.

It's okay to switch it up! If you're looking to get ready for a family vacation or an important event, try high-intensity exercise during non-fasting periods. Your body needs fuel, and while there are benefits to working out while fasting, save your brand-new hot yoga class for a later time.

That's the beauty of intermittent fasting: You choose what you do and when!

Lastly, keep yourself hydrated. Check back to the last chapter if you need a refresher. Electrolyte imbalances are no joke. If your electrolytes are out of wack, you might feel nauseous, dizzy, crampy, and achy. Use the drinks and liquids I introduced to avoid unnecessary discomfort.

Planning Your Routine

In general, there are two exercise categories: aerobic and anaerobic.

Aerobic exercise (think back to your 80s aerobics class) is a long-term form of workout. Running, walking, cycling, and other long-term activities (usually more than thirty minutes) are aerobic exercises. If you're exercising on an empty stomach or during a fast, stick to aerobic exercises.

Aerobic exercises are what professionals call "easy cardio." Easy cardio doesn't include running; in fact, long-term running isn't recommended during a fast. If you're an avid runner, stick to short, low intensity running sprints if you're exercising during a fast.

Stick to the "aerobic zone," or the heart rate zone where your body burns the most fat. This may seem a little contradictory but staying within the area best for your heart health keeps your body engaged and hydrated.

Scientists theorize that most people "should be able to remain active in that zone almost indefinitely without needing much, or any, food" (Sisson, 2020).

If you're a little confused about this range, don't worry. I'll show you how to calculate your ideal aerobic zone. Keep in mind that there are different ways to calculate your ideal heart rate zone. I've found this method to be the most accurate (and easiest to calculate!).

First, subtract your age in years from 220.

So, if you're 50 years old, your number would be 170 heartbeats per minute.

Let's do some more math. Multiply this number by 64% for your bottom rate, and 76% for your top heart rate.

170 x 0.64= 109 beats per minute

170 x 0.76= 129 beats per minute

So again, if you're 50 years old, your target aerobic heart rate is between 109 and 129 heartbeats per minute.

You don't need an expensive heart rate monitor, though, for some people, these are quite helpful. Listen to your body; you shouldn't feel overexerted if you're within your target heart rate. Your target heart rate range is the space where your body isn't dipping too far into your glycogen stores. In this range, you're burning fat!

Anaerobic exercises include sprinting, high-intensity interval training (HIIT) workouts, or heavy weightlifting. It's a short-term form of exercise that requires a great deal of effort.

The anaerobic heart rate zone calculations work similarly to the ones we tried before, except the percentages are a bit higher.

Subtract your age from 220 again; if you're fifty years old, this number is 170 heartbeats per minute.

Then, multiply this number by 80% and 90% respectively.

170 x 0.8= 136 beats per minute

170 X 0.9= 153 beats per minute

So, if you are fifty years old, your anaerobic heart rate zone is between 136 and 153.

It's okay to engage in anaerobic exercises but be sure to fuel up before or after hitting the gym or track. Scientists don't recommend engaging in high-intensity, anaerobic exercises during a fast.

I'm not saying you should completely avoid hitting your anaerobic heart rate zone during every workout; it's important to stay conscious.

Eat a healthy meal of protein and complex carbohydrates two or three hours before hitting the gym. Protein helps prepare your muscles for work and gives you the fuel you need to get through your workout.

Protein isn't just for pre-workouts. Consuming protein and healthy fats after a workout help your body recover. If you don't fully recover, your workouts won't be nearly as effective.

Give your body the fuel it needs.

Finally, listen to your body. If you're a self-proclaimed fitness nut, you might notice some changes in your body during a fasted workout. It's okay; don't panic. Your body needs time. If you're new to the exercise game, take it slow and low.

You can do this.

Yoga: The Faster's Crash Course

You might be a yoga fanatic or a yoga newbie; regardless, yoga and intermittent fasting go hand-in-hand. Yoga is a spiritual practice as much as it is a healthy one, just like intermittent fasting.

Certain forms of yoga are more high intensity than others (think hot yoga), but, as a whole, yoga is a fantastic way to reconnect with oneself while improving coordination, and muscle mass, and burning a few calories.

Yoga began as a Hindu spiritual practice. Think back to Chapter 3; intermittent fasting did too! It's a practice rooted in controlled breathing, meditation, and overall health and well-being.

I spoke to Karen A., who told me, "I've been practicing yoga my whole life. I knew about the spiritual benefits, but it wasn't until I turned about 45 that I understood how it would benefit my brain."

If that isn't enough to convince you, let's go a step further to discuss the benefits of practicing yoga.

Improved Strength and Balance

Most don't think of strength when they think of yoga; you might consider weightlifting, cycling, etc. If this is your initial assumption, keep reading.

Yoga promotes increased blood flow to your muscles. It provides them necessary oxygen to recoup and rejuvenate. Studies show that "yoga [is] an effective strength-building practice across many age groups" (Link, 2017).

Yoga stabilizes your core, allowing you to build your abdominal muscles and support your organs. It's also a great way to improve muscle tone, particularly in your arms and legs.

Yoga improves balance. As we age, our balancing skills take a hit. You might not be interested in sitting on your head or balancing on one leg, but balance and coordination prevent certain accidents that can complicate your overall health.

Regardless of your yoga skill level, all yoga positions, when practiced safely, improve balance, flexibility, and bodily strength.

Improved Flexibility

This one may seem like a given: Yoga positively affects flexibility through a series of semi-strenuous, structured movements held over long periods.

We still haven't answered the question: Why is flexibility important? You might not be looking to try a middle split anytime soon, so why should you care about flexibility?

Flexibility improves coordination and aids in your body's ability to recover from injury. Additionally, yoga changes your body's response to pain. Many people practicing yoga experience less back pain and arthritis symptoms while practicing; scientists believe flexibility is the cause.

We become less flexible as we age. It's natural, but you don't have to fall into this trap. Practicing yoga aids in maintaining flexibility, coordination, and balance as you age.

Age gracefully, my friend.

Yoga and Heart Health

I've talked about heart disease a few times in earlier chapters. Heart disease is an unfortunate reality for many Americans, but it doesn't have to be.

Exercise is known to aid those suffering from heart disease and can also prevent the development of heart blockages and complications; yoga goes a step further. Experts believe that yoga might be more effective at decreasing the rates of heart disease compared to normal modes of working out.

Yoga is relaxing for both the body and mind. Over time, mental and emotional stress can increase your body's production of cortisol, "which narrow[s] your arteries and increase blood pressure" (*The Yoga-Heart Connection*, 2019).

Yoga utilizes a term called, pranayama, otherwise known as yoga breathing. Many studies show a link between pranayama and improved cardiovascular functioning.

Your heart loves controlled breathing. Those practicing yoga enjoy "favorable changes in heart rate, stroke capacity, arterial pressure, and contractility of the heart" (Link, 2017).

Studies show that yoga is a great tool to lower blood glucose levels and resting heart rate, which prevents both the onset of heart disease and type 2 diabetes. It's also shown to benefit weight loss: Those practicing yoga enjoy a smaller waist circumference than those who don't.

Long story short, it works pretty well!

Trouble Falling Asleep? Try Yoga

Yoga is relaxing. It's a great way to wind down after a day of errands, plans, and stressful meetings.

Menopause causes certain changes in our sleep patterns, none of which are favorable. Yoga provides certain calming effects: Your body positively releases stress, leading to a better, more restful night's sleep.

Studies back it up; some studies indicate that yoga is a particularly effective holistic method to regulate sleep patterns.

Yoga and Self-Esteem

Some people, including myself, struggle with body image issues. I feel most people do. We're not happy when we look in the mirror, or, if we are, we still find areas or parts of our bodies we'd like to change.

But just because it's a widespread belief doesn't mean it's okay, nor should it be 'normal.'

Yoga is relaxing. We know that much already. But yoga yields some pretty amazing mental benefits that last beyond your 3 PM Savasana class.

Yoga is a means of stress reduction; studies show a positive correlation when comparing those practicing yoga and perceived body image. Yoga contributes to lower incidences of depression and improved symptoms, particularly in those struggling with body image.

It goes a bit beyond self-esteem. If you struggle with low self-esteem, you might also notice changes in your quality of life. I had damaging self-esteem issues in my forties; I felt disgruntled and uncomfortable. These issues didn't go away when I entered menopause. I struggled to leave the house, spend time with family, and engage in meaningful, positive thinking.

In short, my quality of life suffered.

The term quality of life refers to your unique perception of the world around you. It refers to the way you interact with the world concerning your personal goals and expectations.

Your "relationships, creativity, learning opportunities, health, and material comforts" can positively or negatively affect your quality of life (Link, 2017).

Yoga allows its proponents to gain a better understanding of their body: They understand how it moves, why it moves, and learn how to move in a way that provides relaxation.

While the cause of this correlation is unknown, studies show a positive relationship between yoga enthusiasts and a positive outlook.

Yoga and Mental Health

Practicing yoga is linked to decreased symptoms of depression and anxiety; it's considered a holistic method of symptom management.

No one *enjoys* being stressed. At least, most people don't. I fall into the latter category.

Stress is a powerful motivator: You're more productive when facing a deadline or when you have a set series of daily tasks. Stress becomes a problem when it becomes negative.

Many women report negative stress during menopause. I felt this phenomenon firsthand. Negative stress contributes to a negative outlook. Those suffering from constant, intrusive thoughts are dealing with negative stress. If you struggle to fall asleep, feel consistently exhausted, and feel overwhelmed daily, you might be suffering from negative stress.

Mental health professionals believe anxiety, otherwise known as generalized anxiety disorder, is the most common mental health disorder in the U.S.

Studies suggest that yoga "may be effective as an alternative treatment for anxiety disorders" (Link, 2017). The act of checking in with oneself, even for an hour, improves your attitude toward life.

Depression is another common mental illness, and for many, it's debilitating. Depression isn't sadness or dismay; those suffering from depression feel constant dissatisfaction and emptiness. Some report not being able to get out of bed and thoughts of suicide.

While yoga can't cure depression, it might help. One 2017 study "[looked] at the effects of yoga-based treatments on depressive symptoms overwhelmingly concluded that yoga can now be considered an effective alternative treatment" for those suffering from depression (Link, 2017).

Yoga and Menopause: Why and How

Hot flashes, sleep disturbances, anxiety, depression, and changes in appetite are common symptoms of menopause. You might feel confused, frustrated, or anguished. The point is—many women experience these symptoms, and some of those women use yoga to cope.

Many women have found that yoga, including restorative and supportive poses, may improve the undesirable side effects of menopause.

That's where restorative yoga comes in. Those practicing restorative yoga hold poses longer than those practicing other schools of yoga; they use blankets and other props to guide their movements and support their body.

Let's introduce some yoga poses you can try when you're feeling menopausal symptoms. I'll use the English labels for these poses for your understanding.

Reclining Bound Angle Pose

This one is a little easier, so if you're a beginner yogi, start here!

Begin sitting up on the mat and stretch your legs out in front of you. Bend both knees and keep them on the floor. Bring your feet together to form a square shape.

Lean back and lay on the mat. Maintain the square shape. If you need support, press your palms into your mat. Lay as flat as possible.

Maintain this pose for five to ten minutes.

Release any tension with relaxed breaths. Closing your eyes may help. Feel your chest move up and down and relax when you decide to sit up.

The reclining bound angle pose is effective for those struggling with fatigue, tight legs, and stress.

Shoulder Stand

Begin lying down on a mat or the floor. Your back should be flat against the ground. Next, use a wall and straighten your legs against it. Position them up in the air. Hold this pose for a few seconds.

Flex your toes and move your legs away from the wall. Support them with your muscles.

Now, hold the pose for about a minute. Inhale and exhale a few times (aim for about eight) before bringing your feet down with your final exhale.

Some prefer to try a more advanced form of the shoulder stand: Put your body in a bridge pose and lift your hips off the mat. Keep your palms down by your sides and lift your legs in the air, straightening them as much as possible. Some prefer to place their palms under the arch of their back for support.

The only difference between the two forms is the wall; begin with the first method before advancing.

This pose brings clarity, stress relief, muscle strengthening, and digestive benefits. However, if you suffer from a neck or back injury, take caution.

Reclining Hero Pose

This one is pretty simple too!

Begin sitting up straight on your mat; keep both feet and legs in line with your hips and flat on the mat. If you're a beginner yoga master, you can use a rolled-up blanket, pillow, chair, or cushion to support your back and bottom throughout the pose. Personally, I find the pillow the most comfortable!

You have two options for this pose, and I'll explain both!

If you're new to yoga, try the pose with one leg. Slide one foot (left or right, it doesn't matter) towards the outer side of your thigh. Form a diamond in that direction. If you're comfortable, touch your calf to that thigh. If not, a little distance is okay too! After about 10-20 seconds, relax your leg and do the same with the other.

If you're an avid yogi, try doing the same with both legs at once. This is relatively difficult, so don't over-exert yourself!

Lean back carefully and use your elbows and arms to support the pose while you're doing either of these versions. Use the pillow to support your positioning.

Breathe deeply and focus on how your legs feel. If you feel uncomfortable or strained, relax the pose. Inhale and exhale throughout.

When you're done, use your arms and the pillow or cushion to guide yourself back to a sitting position.

This pose is great for leg and abdomen flexibility and can improve digestion. If you suffer from chronic leg or knee pain, or recently had knee surgery, skip this one!

Mariachi's Pose

You'll need a belt, rope, or cord for this one. Sit on your mat with your legs stretched out and flat on the floor. Ensure your legs are parallel with each hip. Flex your toes and bend one knee; place your foot on the floor.

Use a belt, cord, or strap, and use the arm adjacent to the leg you bent to reach around your back. Move your other arm around your back as well and hold the strap tightly. If you can't touch your arms together, that's okay! Leave a few inches of the strap between your hands. Don't strain your arm muscles.

Hold for up to one minute and breathe deeply. Relax your arms slowly, and exhale as you break the pose.

Mariachi's pose slows your breath and stretches your back and shoulders. Some believe this pose improves digestion, but regardless, give it a try.

Head-to-Knee Forward Bend

You'll need a strap for this pose as well. Sit on your mat and stretch your legs in front of you. Keep them in line with your hips. Bend one knee and place the foot on the floor, similar to the last pose.

Keep your abdomen centered and bend at the waist, leaning over as though to touch the leg remaining on the floor. Position the strap around that foot and use it to support your stretch. Use as many or as little strap as you need to guide your movement.

Hold for as long as you can; aim for one minute. Inhale and exhale out of the pose.

This pose benefits your spine and relieves anxiety and headaches. However, if you suffer from chronic back pain, avoid this pose.

Downward-Facing Dog

This is a popular pose, and you're likely relatively familiar. If not, I'm going to go through it!

Start on your hands and knees (like a dog!) and align your hips with your shoulders. Stretch your legs and form a bridge shape; press your feet to the floor. It might feel difficult to use your whole foot, so if you need to start on your toes or the balls of your feet, that's okay.

If you look like a bridge, you're almost there. Drop your head and focus on your alignment.

Hold the pose for about ten seconds; sway a bit if you need to. When you're done, lower your knees and use them to release your arms from the floor or mat.

This pose strengthens your arm and leg muscles, relaxes your back, and enhances your breathing.

Bridge Pose

You looked a bit like a bridge in the downward dog, but in this pose, you'll use your legs to form a bridge. They do the work, not your arms.

Lie flat on your back. Ensure your whole body is flat, including your legs. Place your palms on the mat next to you and bend your knees. Press your feet to the floor beneath you. Your feet should be relatively close to your bottom, but this takes practice.

Continue pressing your feet to the floor and use them to push your hips up, forming a sort of triangle.

Place your palms under the arch of your back and use them to support the pose. Hold the pose for thirty seconds. When you're done, release your back and place your bottom on the floor.

The bridge pose is effective for those struggling with mild depression, anxiety, digestive issues, and stress. It's a great way to relieve back pain and encourages mental clarity.

Always consult a professional before trying these poses. If you need more guidance, don't be afraid to check out links and videos online.

Don't overdo it, at least, not at first. Yoga, just like intermittent fasting, is a practice. It's not easy, but with proper habits, you'll be a yogi pro in no time.

Fun Ways to Move

Maybe yoga isn't for you. Perhaps you had a particularly traumatic experience with a bicycle a few years ago. Maybe you just don't like exercising.

That's okay!

Here are some less-discussed ways you can start exercising today.

- Roller Skating
- Hiking
- Kayaking
- At-home exercise videos
- Bodyweight movements with cans, books, or household items
- Dancing (Zumba, Barre, or just dancing around your space!)
- Jumping rope
- Swimming

- Golf
- Martial arts

And that's simply to name a few. However, some of those exercises require time, effort, and skill. Rigid, formulaic exercise routines aren't for everyone, and gym memberships can cost a pretty penny depending on where you live. So, how can you get out there and move a little without balance, a gym, or a kayak? Here are some exercise hacks.

- Exploring your town or city
- Cleaning your living space (really get into those nooks and crannies)
- Babysitting children
- Walking to lunch
- Using a standing or convertible desk
- Playing a fun video game (Wii is a great example)

Again, these are simply a few examples. Try exercises that feel right for you. Get creative!

Move Forward

You don't need to buy a gym membership or an expensive free weight rack to get moving. Most people don't need either of these at all!

Exercise is a somewhat polarizing topic: Some people rave about it while others shy away, rejecting the topic altogether. I fell into the latter category for a long time. I can relate.

Exercising and getting out there is a bit daunting, especially if it's been a while since you hit the gym. That's okay. There's nothing to be afraid of.

Hold yourself accountable and remain conscious. If you're lethargic one day, skip your walk. If you're especially energetic the next, dance around your space.

Intermittent fasting and exercise go hand-in-hand. You choose how and when you fast; you choose when and how you get movin'.

Chapter 6:
Perimenopause Food and Fasting Plan

"As a physician who knows the importance of body image to our overall health, I wanted to have a way to inspire women to love their bodies no matter what size or shape they are. This is possible! And I know exactly how to do this because I've done it myself, and I've helped thousands of others to do the same thing. It's women's health at its most fundamental level!"

— **Christiane Northrup**

We've discussed the basics. We know the steps. We understand the benefits. I haven't gone into depth about menopause and intermittent fasting. You might be a bit confused as to why we haven't gone through it yet. Don't worry. Keep reading.

Menopause is a reality. I'll be the first to tell you that it's not fun or exciting. It's daunting, and few (if any) women look forward to it.

Luckily, there are many ways to cope with menopause symptoms. If you're thinking about diet and intermittent fasting, you're correct.

In this Chapter, I'll discuss perimenopause, and its symptoms, and introduce a five-day diet plan to mitigate your menopause worries.

What Is Menopause?

Menopause is a natural, biological process that occurs when women reach their late 40s and 50s. Most women in the United States report perimenopause beginning around the age of 45, but this number varies depending on lifestyle, genetic, and cultural factors.

Additionally, women who have gone through an oophorectomy, hysterectomy, or, in some cases, a mastectomy might trigger menopause.

Other surgeries can cause menopause too; my own mother fell into this category. She suffered from colon cancer when I was a girl—she wasn't older than 45. We have a family history of colon cancer, and while the doctor said she "should've been prepared," she was anything but.

Physicians were able to surgically remove cancer, so she didn't have to endure chemotherapy, but the surgery ended up triggering menopause, which caused a host of other issues.

Not only was she frustrated, angry, depressed, and anxious, she had hot flashes to deal with.

Many women fall into this unfortunate boat; this book is here to help.

During and leading up to menopause, your body changes. You metabolize food and glucose less efficiently, LDL cholesterol, or bad cholesterol, levels increase, HDL levels (good cholesterol) decrease, muscle mass declines, your hormone levels fluctuate, and most women report gaining weight.

In short, it's a pretty big transition.

These bodily changes trigger many symptoms, like vaginal dryness, chills, hot flashes, sleep disruptions, changes in mood, weight gain, thinning hair, and even acne.

Menopause occurs in three stages perimenopause, mid-menopause, and post-menopause. Overall, menopause lasts between three and ten years, but post-menopause lasts for the rest of your life.

I don't want you to panic, but you deserve to know the facts.

Perimenopause: What, Why, and Is It Happening to you?

Perimenopause refers to the start of these symptoms; it's the precursor to full-blown menopause. Perimenopause can last between one and five years, though most women report it lasting toward the lower end of that estimate.

Your body is preparing for the transition, and it's not comfortable.

During perimenopause, your ovaries stop working. They no longer release eggs, and, if they do, the frequency becomes irregular. Your body produces less estrogen than it is used to and you slowly lose fertility.

So what happens? How do symptoms arise? What's really going on?

A lot.

As your ovaries stop releasing eggs, you'll notice irregular periods. Some women report much longer periods, but it varies from person to person. Over time, your periods will dwindle; eventually, you won't have them at all.

During perimenopause, you'll experience hot flashes. It's thought that hot flashes are related to changes in your estrogen levels; you might feel a sudden warm feeling, or your face might become flushed. Some women don't experience hot flashes at all, while others have strong hot flashes lasting for over ten minutes.

No one enjoys them, so instead of getting frustrated, try cooling food! Foods like apples, eggs, tea, spinach, and bananas can help your body quickly recover from hot flashes.

I've included recipes for delicious meals that contain each of these menopause-healthy foods!

You might feel more frustrated or irritable around menopause; it's to be expected. Scientists aren't certain what causes menopausal irritability. Some theorize that life simply becomes more complicated as we grow older, while others believe that estrogen levels are the cause. While intermittent fasting can't completely remedy depression or severe anxiety, mindfulness practices can help you cope with mood changes.

As your hormone levels change, so does your metabolism. Your body will adjust: You might hold fat in your stomach or upper thighs, and you might lose muscle. Most women report weight gain during perimenopause. It's frustrating, angering even. Some women feel out of touch with their bodies; the lack of control can feel insufferable.

That's where intermittent fasting and healthy eating come into play. Don't lose yourself. Learn how to move forward.

There is hope.

The Perimenopause Diet

There's a direct link between what we eat and how we feel. Food fuels your body and regulates hormone levels, metabolism, and muscle mass.

While food can't reverse menopause, eating certain food groups, coupled with intermittent fasting, can mitigate some of the unfortunate symptoms that accompany this new life change.

Plant-Based Foods

You don't have to go full-blown vegan or vegetarian to alleviate some of the symptoms of perimenopause. Incorporating healthy, plant-based foods into your non fast meals can help reduce the rate of hot flashes.

Scientists report a strong link between a plant-based diet and physical and mental health. We all want to feel healthier and more alert, right?

Recommendations vary depending on where you look: the CDC recommends all adults eat two servings and recommend between two and three vegetable servings daily to reap the full benefits of fruit and veggies, while the AHA recommends four to five servings of each. You really can't go too overboard with fruits and vegetables, so we'll base our recommendations on the AHA guidelines.

But again, you can get creative! One fruit serving looks like a medium piece of fruit (apples, plums, oranges, etc.), a quarter cup of your fruit juice of choice, or a half cup of canned or frozen fruit. One vegetable serving could be three ounces of carrots, one cup of a leafy green (spinach, lettuce, or kale), or half a cup of vegetable juice.

Bring fruit with you as a snack throughout the day or use it to break a fast and try using spinach for salads or cooking.

Follow a diverse diet filled with beneficial minerals and nutrients. Eat vegetables, colorful fruits, and lean protein products.

Fiber

Fiber is pretty important, especially for intermittent fasters. Most people don't eat enough fiber; it's a nutrient that provides fullness, aids in digestion, lowers rates of depression, and improves muscle strength.

Fiber is the carb that isn't; while other carbohydrates, complex or simple, pass through the digestive tract, fiber doesn't. Fiber remains intact throughout your body systems, while the digestive system breaks down other carbohydrates for energy.

The greatest benefit of consuming more fiber is fullness! Feeling full and satisfied is important for anyone, but especially those practicing intermittent fasting. If you feel full during your non-fasting period, you're more likely to stay fuller longer, throughout your fast!

Fiber is sometimes called bulk, but don't let that scare you! Fiber won't bulk you up in any way; in fact, fiber plays an important role in both weight management and blood sugar levels. And, even more, people who consume plenty of fiber are at lower risk of heart disease, and cancer, and tend to live longer than their counterparts!

The Dietary Guidelines for Americans dictate that women under the age of fifty should aim to eat about 25 grams of fiber per day, and women over fifty should consume about 21 grams of fiber per day.

Getting enough fiber isn't too hard, you just need to know where to look! For example, 1 cup of raspberries contains about nine grams of fiber, a medium apple contains almost 5 grams, and one cup of green peas contains nine too! One cup of whole wheat spaghetti contains 6 grams of fiber and 1 cup of brown rice contains another 3.5 grams.

If you're a fifty-one-year-old woman, all you need is an apple with lunch and whole wheat spaghetti with healthy tomato sauce and peas for dinner.

This is just an example. There are many ways you can hit your fiber goals with ease!

Fruits, veggies, whole grain products, and beans are great sources of fiber and go hand-in-hand with a healthy diet, regardless of your age.

Vitamins and Minerals

Many women report feeling weaker during perimenopause and vitamins and minerals are here to help. Additionally, as we age, our bones take a hit. Many women receiving inadequate nutrients develop osteoporosis, which can lead to low recovery time and broken bones if left untreated.

Vitamins and minerals like calcium, magnesium, vitamin C, and vitamin E, are all important, especially during perimenopause.

Think back to Health class—low-fat dairy products are great sources of calcium. But they're not your only option. In other words, if you don't eat dairy products, you're in luck!

Calcium guidelines vary depending on where you look, but women in menopause should aim to consume between 1000 and 1200 mg of calcium per day. That sounds like a lot, but you have plenty of options!

One cup of skim milk contains about 300 mg of calcium, and calcium-fortified soy milk contains up to 400 mg! One ounce of hard cheeses like cheddar and mozzarella contains about 200 mg of calcium as well.

If you're not a dairy person, don't fear! One cup of arugula contains 125 mg of calcium, 1 cup of spinach contains 240 mg, calcium-fortified orange juice contains 300 mg, and half a cup of calcium-fortified cereal contains 250 mg of calcium.

So, if you break a fast or start your day with cereal and soy milk, followed by orange juice and a spinach salad, you're good to go!

Magnesium isn't as prominent, but it's no less important. Again, guidelines vary a bit, but women over fifty should aim for 320 mg of magnesium a day.

You have options! One ounce of dark chocolate contains 64 mg of magnesium, half a cup of spinach contains about 78 mg, and 1 cup of plain yogurt offers another 42 mg. Half a cup of quinoa and half a cup of black beans both contain about 60 mg, and one ounce of roasted pumpkin seeds contains up to 150 mg of magnesium.

Again, if you eat a spinach salad with black beans, roasted pumpkin seeds, and some dark chocolate for dessert, you're on track!

Vitamin C and vitamin E are powerful antioxidants; both also aid in bone and muscle health.

The Recommended Dietary Allowance (RDA) for vitamin C in women is around 75 mg for women and the RDA for vitamin E is 15 mg.

One yellow pepper offers over 300 mg of vitamin C, and 3.5 grams of kale contains another 93 mg! For vitamin E, one ounce of sunflower seeds boasts 10 mg of vitamin E, one ounce of almonds contains about 7 mg, seven ounces of salmon offers 2 mg, and one red pepper contains over 2 mg.

If you have a kale salad with sunflower seeds and almonds, followed by a chopped pepper meal with roasted salmon, you've already hit your goals!

It sounds like a lot of information, so here's a hack: Try colorful foods. Each of the foods I noted was all sorts of colors, like green, red, yellow, and brown.

Make your plate a rainbow!

Omega-3 Fatty Acids

Salmon and mackerel contain powerful omega-3 fatty acids that improve your heart health. Studies point to a link between omega-3 fatty acids and lower incidents of night sweats and mood changes, especially in perimenopausal women.

Omega-3 fatty acid recommendations vary, but most sources recommend eating about 2 grams of healthy fatty acids daily.

Three grams of salmon contains over 2,150 mg of omega-3 fatty acids, and flaxseed contains another 2,350 mg.

I'm not saying you should load up on salmon daily; choose omega-3-rich foods you like and enjoy!

How to Eat Like a Perimenopause Intermittent Fasting Pro

It's easier said than done. But you're in luck. Intermittent fasting and healthy eating go hand in hand; what you eat outside of your fast is nearly as important as the fast itself!

I'll introduce a five-day meal plan with recipes to help you begin your perimenopause journey. This might seem a bit counterintuitive: Why is a book about fasting discussing recipes?

We discussed the importance of what you eat versus when you choose not to in the earlier chapters. Each of these recipes contains important fast-breaking and fast-sustaining ingredients like fiber, veggies, and fruits to keep you full throughout the day!

Not only that—I've included a few recipes to help you maintain a prolonged fast; think the 5:2 method! Scientists recommend "[breaking] a fast with a nourishing soup and some cooked veggies because they are easier to digest and absorb," (Eckelkamp, 2020). Apple crumble, avocado and eggs, and the Moroccan eggplant recipes are all permissible during a 5:2 fast. Choose healthy recipes that interest you!

Pick recipes that work within your intermittent fasting schedule.

Breakfast

Banana Pancakes (Vegetarian & Gluten-Free)

Prep time: 10 minutes

Cook time: 5-7 minutes

Total: 15-17 minutes

Ingredients

½ cup oats

1 tablespoon coconut flour (almond or normal flour work as well)

¼ unsweetened almond milk (cow milk may also be used)

¼ cup fat-free Greek Yogurt

1 banana

2 teaspoons baking powder

1 scoop protein powder (vanilla works best)

2 egg whites

¼ teaspoon ground cinnamon

Instructions

1. Use a food processor to grind the oats until smooth.

2. Add the yogurt, flour, milk of choice, extract, egg whites, cinnamon, half of the banana, baking powder, and protein powder. Process until well combined.

3. Preheat a large skillet over medium heat and spray with cooking spray. Pour about a ⅓ cup of batter into the pan and cook for 3-4 minutes on each side. If you'd like larger pancakes, use ½ cup of batter and cook for an extra minute.

4. Top with slices of the remaining half banana.

Nutrition Information

Calories: 163, Carbohydrates: 31 g, Fiber: 2 g, Protein: 9 g, Fat: 1 g

Apple Crumble: A Breakfast Take on a Classic (Vegan & Gluten-Free)

Prep Time: 10 -12 minutes

Cook Time: 30-40 minutes

Total Time: 50 minutes to an hour

Ingredients

6 large red apples

2 teaspoons and 1 tablespoon coconut oil (butter substitute is okay, but isn't recommended)

1 tbsp cinnamon

⅔ cup of pecans (almonds work as well)

⅔ cup oats

2 teaspoons honey

Instructions

1. Cut the apples into wedges and add them to a large saucepan. Add 2 teaspoons coconut oil and cinnamon. Sauté over medium-high heat for 5 minutes. Cover for a few minutes until the apples are soft.

2. Preheat the oven to 350 degrees (375 degrees for a crisper taste).

3. Add the nuts, oats, remaining coconut oil, and honey to a food processor and pulse until the mixture begins to stick together a bit.

4. Use a rectangular cake pan or cookie sheet and lay the apples flat. Top with the crumble.

5. Bake for 15 minutes.

Note: Try the recipe with yogurt or honey drizzle for a more fulfilling meal!

Nutrition Information

(For ½ cup serving)

Calories: 380, Carbohydrates: 54 g, Fiber: 11 g, Protein: 4 g, Fat: 20 g

Carrot Cake Oats (Vegan & Gluten-Free)

Prep Time: 10 minutes

Cook Time: 0 minutes

Total Time: 10 minutes

Ingredients

1 cup oats

½ cup shredded carrot

1 teaspoon cinnamon

¼ teaspoon allspice (this may be left out at your discretion)

3 tablespoons raisins

1 tablespoon chia seeds

1 teaspoon vanilla extract

3 tablespoons maple syrup

1 ¼ cup of unsweetened almond milk

1. Combine the oats, carrots, cinnamon, allspice, raisins, and chia seeds in a large mixing bowl.

2. Add vanilla, syrup, and almond milk.

3. Place in small ramekins or leave in a bowl at your leisure. Refrigerate overnight.

4. Add pecans, almonds, or your nuts of choice!

Nutrition Information

(For ½ of the recipe)

Calories: 340, Carbohydrates: 70 g, Fiber: 9 g, Protein: 8 g, Fat: 4 g

Avocado & Eggs (Vegetarian & Gluten-Free)

Prep Time: 10 mins

Cook Time: 15 mins

Total Time: 25 mins

Ingredients

1 ripe Haas avocado

2 eggs

Pinch of salt

Pinch of ground pepper

Red pepper flakes (optional)

Parsley if desired

Instructions

1. Begin preheating the oven to 450 degrees. Line a baking sheet with foil.

2. Cut the avocado in half and remove the pit. Scoop out the avocado meat and save for another recipe!

3. Crack eggs in a separate bowl and whisk. You can separate the yolk if you're looking for more of a poached egg, but scrambled is my preferred style.

4. Season with salt, pepper, and red pepper flakes.

5. Bake for about 15 minutes to your desired doneness.

6. Let them cool down and enjoy!

Nutrition Information

Calories: 208

Carbohydrates: 8 g, Fiber: 6 g, Protein: 7 g, Fat: 17 g

Berry Yogurt Parfait (Vegetarian & Gluten-Free)

Prep time: 5 minutes

Cook time: 0 minutes

Total time: 5 minutes

Ingredients

1 cup of unsweetened Greek yogurt

½ cup mixed berries (I prefer blueberries and strawberries)

You may also add sliced almonds or granola

Instructions

1. Add the yogurt to a cup, ramekin, mason jar, or bowl of choice

2. Add the berries and optional toppings.

3. Enjoy!

Nutrition Information

Calories: 194 calories, Carbohydrates: 14 g, Fiber: 1 g, Protein: 23 g, Fat: 4 g

Lunch

Instant Noodle Pot

Prep time: 10 minutes

Cook Time: 5 minutes

Total Time: 15 minutes

Ingredients

½ Rice Noodle Nest (pre-cooked)

½ of a chicken breast (pre-shredded)

2 Bak Choi leaves

Grated carrot to your liking

A few tablespoons of grated ginger

1 small broth cube

2 teaspoons soy sauce

¼ cup chopped yellow onion

½ cup chopped spinach

4 sugar snap peas

1 cup chopped red bell pepper

Instructions

1. Collect a few mason jars and add the cooked noodles to the bottom of each jar. Add the pre-shredded chicken and ginger.

2. Make the stock from the package instructions and pour it over the noodles. Add soy sauce.

3. Add peppers, Bak Choi, spinach, onion, carrot, and peas to the jar.

4. Refrigerate for at least an hour.

5. When you're ready to eat, add boiling water and let sit for about three minutes.

6. Enjoy!

Note: If you'd like to boost the protein in the recipe, add some chopped tofu!

Nutrition Information

(For 1 serving)

Calories: 522 , Carbohydrate: 82 g, Fiber: 13 g, Protein: 40 g, Fat: 5 g

Avocado Shrimp Salad (Pescatarian & Gluten-Free)

Prep time: 5 minutes

Cook time: 10 minutes

Total time: 15 minutes

Ingredients

1 lb. shrimp

1 and 3 tablespoons extra virgin olive oil

2 avocados (pre-peeled)

Salt and pepper to taste

3 tablespoons red onion

1 tablespoon cilantro

1 ½ cups of shredded lettuce

Lime juice

Instructions

1. Steam the shrimp. Bring a large pot of water to a continuous, rolling boil. Add your shrimp into a mesh strainer and steam over the pot until pink.

2. Add shrimp to a bowl. Add olive oil, salt and pepper, red onion, cilantro, and lettuce. Stir to combine.

3. Make the dressing. Add the olive oil and lemon juice to a small mixing bowl and whisk for a bit.

4. Add the dressing to the salad. Slice the avocados and add to the top!

Note: Serve the recipe on whole-grain bread for a serving of healthy carbohydrates.

Nutrition Information

Calories: 363, Carbohydrates: 7 g, Fiber: 5 g, Protein: 24 g, Fat: 26 g

Not Your Campbell's Tomato Soup (Vegetarian & Gluten-Free)

Prep time: 10 minutes

Cook time: 25 minutes

Total time: 35 minutes

Ingredients

2 lbs. of Roma tomatoes

2 tablespoons of extra-virgin olive oil

1 white onion

2 teaspoons garlic, minced

1 ½ cups chicken broth

⅓ cup plain Greek yogurt (no flavoring)

1 tablespoon fresh basil

¼ cup cornstarch

Salt and pepper to taste

Instructions

1. Boil water over medium-high heat in a large pot. Once boiling, add tomatoes and leave in the pot until the skin begins to crack. Remove the tomatoes and let them cool for a bit.

2. Chop the onion and add to a separate pot with the olive oil. Let it cook over medium heat. Add the garlic and sauté for a few minutes.

3. Remove the tomato skin and chop the tomatoes. Add them to a blender with the onions, vegetable broth, yogurt, salt and pepper, and basil. Blend until nice and smooth.

4. Add everything back to the pot and simmer over medium-low heat.

5. In another small mixing bowl, whisk the cornstarch and water until thickened. Add the mixture, but by bit, to the pot and stir vigorously until thick. You might not use all of the corn starch mixtures.

6. Enjoy!

Note: Serve with whole wheat bread if desired.

Nutrition Information

(For 1 cup serving)

Calories: 135, Carbohydrates: 16 g, Fiber: 3 g, Protein: 5 g, Fat: 6 g

Yummy Taco Salad

Prep time: 20 minutes

Cook time: 10-15 minutes

Total time: 30-35 minutes

Ingredients

2 small flour tortillas

2 teaspoons extra-virgin olive oil

Salt and pepper to taste

1 pound of lean ground turkey

1 tablespoon of chili powder

1 teaspoon of ground cumin

½ teaspoon garlic powder

1 head of romaine lettuce, chopped

1 can of reduced-sodium black beans, pre drained

1 can of corn, drained

2 cups of halved cherry tomatoes

1 ripe avocado, diced

1 cup of cilantro leaves pre-chopped

½ cup reduced-fat shredded sharp cheddar cheese

¼ cup green onions

½ cup salsa of choice

½ cup greek yogurt (unflavored)

Instructions

1. Preheat your oven to 425 degrees F.

2. Cut each tortilla into strips. Add onto a baking sheet (with cooking spray) and drizzle on the olive oil and some salt and pepper. Coat the tortillas with the oil. Bake for about 9 minutes.

3. Add a bit of olive oil to a large pot and heat over medium. Add the turkey, cumin, garlic powder, chili powder, and some more salt and pepper. Cook the meat mixture.

4. Next, whisk together the salsa and yogurt.

5. Add the lettuce to a bowl with the other ingredients. Top with the tortilla strips. Add dressing and stir.

6. You're ready to eat!

Note: Use whole grain tortillas for an extra kick of complex carbohydrates.

Nutrition Information

(For 1 medium serving without the dressing)

Calories: 596, Carbohydrates: 65 g, Fiber: 18 g, Protein: 40 g, Fat: 23 g

Dinner

Pesto Pea Pasta (Vegan & Gluten-Free)

Prep time: 15 minutes

Cook time: 15 minutes

Total time: 30 minutes

Ingredients

1 ½ cups basil

½ cup of chopped parsley

1 cup of green peas

2 tablespoons of garlic

¼ cup of pine nuts

2 tablespoons of lemon juice

¼ cup vegan parmesan cheese

Sea salt to taste

¼ cup of extra-virgin olive oil

10 ounces of gluten-free pasta

An extra 1 tablespoon of extra-virgin olive oil

2 cloves of garlic (pre-chopped)

1 cup of arugula

¼ cup of sun-dried tomatoes

Instructions

1. Add water and a bit of salt to a large saucepan and bring to a boil.

2. Use a food processor to thoroughly combine basil, peas, nuts, garlic, olive oil, parsley, cheese, and lemon or lime juice. Keep processing until creamy.

3. Add the pasta to the water pot and cook according to the package directions. Drain the pasta.

4. Grab a separate pot and add olive oil, garlic, and tomatoes. Sauté for a few minutes. Add cooked pasta to the pot and stir to combine.

5. Place the arugula on a separate plate and add some of the pesto. Combine the ingredients.

6. Serve the pasta, arugula, and remaining pesto!

Note: You can keep the pasta for up to two days in the refrigerator. Again, it's a great meal-prepping option!

Nutrition Information

(One serving; recipe serves 4)

Calories: 552, Carbohydrates: 65 g, Fiber: 10 g, Protein: 15 g, Fat: 27 g

Lemon Garlic Chicken Bake (Gluten-Free)

Prep time: 10 minutes

Cook time: 40 minutes

Total time: 50 minutes

Ingredients

4 skinless chicken thighs

10 large carrots

5 small red potatoes

3 cloves of garlic

2 cups green beans

1 lemon

1 sprig thyme

Salt and pepper to taste

Instructions

1. Start by preheating your oven to 400 degrees F.
2. Add some water to a large pan and salt accordingly. Cut the potatoes into small wedges and boil until soft. Take them out and cook the carrots afterward.
3. Grab a roasting pan and spray it with cooking spray. Place the chicken on the roasting tray and season with salt and pepper.
4. Combine potatoes, carrots, garlic, thyme, and lemon (pre-cut and skinned) in a large bowl and stir.
5. Add the potato mixture to the roasting pan with the chicken and cook for thirty minutes or until cooked.
6. Add green beans to the roasting tray after removing them from the oven and place in the oven once more for 10 minutes.
7. Serve!

Note: You can add other vegetables of your choice for a more tailored recipe!

Nutrition Information

(For 1 thigh and a small serving of sides)

Calories: 355, Carbohydrates: 32 g, Protein: 31 g, Fat: 12 g

Parmesan Cod with Zucchini Noodles (Pescatarian & Gluten-Free)

Prep time: 15 minutes

Cook time: 20-25 minutes

Total time: 35-40 minutes

Ingredients

2 medium zucchinis sliced into noodles with a peeler

1 tablespoon coconut oil

1 teaspoon extra-virgin olive oil

Salt and pepper to taste

⅔ cup of grated Parmesan cheese

½ tablespoon of mayonnaise

1 teaspoon of lemon juice

½ teaspoon of dried basil

½ teaspoon of dried oregano

½ teaspoon of onion powder

4 Cod fillets

Instructions

1. Heat the oven to the broil setting (above 450 degrees F).

2. Add zucchini noodles to a large skillet and sauté in olive oil for 5-6 minutes over medium-high heat. Add the salt and pepper to taste.

3. Combine half of the pre-measured parmesan cheese with mayonnaise, basil, oregano, lemon juice, and onion powder. Place your filets on a baking sheet or roasting pan. Top each filet with an equal portion of the parmesan cheese mixture.

4. Broil the filets and toppings for about three minutes. Reduce heat to 320 degrees F and bake for another 5 minutes. Cook until the filets are opaque.

5. Add a quarter of the zucchini pasta to each plate and aff the filet on top. Garnish with the remaining parmesan cheese.

Nutrition Information

(For a 1-cup serving)

Calories: 215, Carbohydrates: 4 g, Fiber: 1 g, Fat: 11 g, Protein: 25 g

Moroccan-Style Eggplant (Vegan & Gluten-Free)

Prep time: 20 minutes

Cook time: 90 minutes

Total time: 1 hour and 50 minutes

Ingredients

2 pounds of eggplant

10 garlic cloves

2 pre-quartered shallots

½ cup extra-virgin olive oil

Salt to taste

2 teaspoons of ras el hanout

1 teaspoon of caraway seeds

Pepper to taste

4 medium pre-quartered Roma tomatoes

1 lemon, zest only

Instructions

1. Preheat your oven to 375 degrees F.
2. Begin cutting the eggplant in half lengthwise and place it on a baking sheet. Add the garlic cloves and shallots.
3. Combine olive oil, salt and pepper, ras el hanout, and seeds in a medium mixing bowl. Pour the mixture over the eggplant and coat well.
4. Cook for about 20 minutes in the oven. Then, lower the heat to about 350 degrees F. Remove from the oven and add tomatoes and lemon zest.
5. Bake for about 75 more minutes and check regularly. Stir each time you check. The eggplant is done when the mixture is creamy.
6. Remove from the oven.

Note: You can add chickpeas for a protein boost.

Nutrition Information

(For 1 serving)

Calories: 219, Carbohydrates: 14 g, Fiber: 5 g, Protein: 3 g, Fat: 19 g

Easy Loaded Sweet Potato Skins (Vegan & Gluten-Free)

Prep time: 25 minutes

Cook time: 80 minutes

Total time: 1 hour and 45 minutes

Ingredients

3 sweet potatoes

2 tablespoons of chopped onion

2 cloves of minced garlic

¼ cup of red bell pepper

¼ cup of diced tomatoes

1 cup of black beans, pre-cooked

2 tablespoons of unsweetened greek yogurt

½ cup of vegan shredded mozzarella cheese (use regular if you're not following a vegan diet)

Salt and pepper to taste

½ teaspoon of paprika

½ of a lime

½ tablespoon of extra-virgin olive oil

Instructions

1. Preheat your oven to 375 degrees F.
2. Use a fork to aerate the sweet potatoes and bake them in the oven for about 45 minutes. Then, slice them in half lengthwise.
3. In a saucepan, add a bit of the olive oil and sauté onion, peppers, garlic, and tomatoes until nice and tender.
4. Scoop out the flesh of your potatoes and add it to a mixing bowl. Combine the sauteed veggies, sweet potato meat, black beans, yogurt, salt and pepper, cheese, and paprika. Stir well.
5. Coat the bottom of the hollow potato skins with the remaining oil and flip them over. Cook for about 10 more minutes.
6. Fill the skins with the veggie mixture and cook for 15 more minutes.
7. Top with lime!

Nutrition Information

(For 1 skin)

Calories: 187, Carbohydrates: 35 g, Fiber: 7 g, Fat: 4 g, Protein: 5 g

Snacks

Not Your Run of the Mill Trail Mix (Can Be Made Vegan & Gluten-Free)

Prep time: 10 minutes

Cook time: 0 minutes

Total time: 10 minutes

Ingredients

1-2 cups assorted raw nuts (you can use almonds, peanuts, etc.)

1 cup of pumpkin seeds

1 cup of unsweetened dried fruit of choice

½ cup chopped extra-dark chocolate*

1 cup unbuttered popcorn*

½ teaspoon sea salt*

Optional ingredients noted with *

Instructions

1. Combine all ingredients in a large mixing bowl and stir until well combined.

2. Store in a sealed container.

3. Enjoy it as a yummy snack!

Note: You can use whatever "add-ins" you like! Pay attention to the fiber and sodium content of your add-ins.

Nutrition facts are not included due to toppings.

Mango Yogurt Parfait (Vegetarian & Gluten-Free)

Prep time: 20 minutes

Cook time: 0 minutes

Total time: 20 minutes

Ingredients

2 large pre-pitted cubed mangos

3 cups low-fat, unsweetened greek yogurt

6 tablespoons of granola

Instructions

1. Add mango to a food processor and puree until smooth. Add an equal amount to six small mason jars or cups.

2. Top with equal amounts of the greek yogurt.

3. Then, top with granola.

4. Refrigerate for 15 minutes and snack accordingly!

Nutrition Information

(For 1 jar or cup)

Calories: 149, Carbohydrates: 28 g, Fiber: 2 g, Protein: 6 g, Fat: 3 g

Easy Roasted Chickpeas (Vegan & Gluten-Free)

Prep time: 5-10 minutes

Cook time: 25 minutes

Total time: 30-35 minutes

Ingredients

1 ½ cups of pre-cooked chickpeas

1 tablespoon of extra-virgin olive oil

Salt to taste

Option spices, including paprika or curry powder

Instructions

1. Preheat your oven to 425 degrees F. Spray a large baking sheet with non-stick cooking spray.

2. Pat the chickpeas dry with a towel and remove the skins accordingly.

3. Spread chickpeas on a baking sheet, drizzle with oil, and season.

4. Bake for 25 minutes.

5. Serve warm.

Nutrition Information

(Per serving size)

Calories: 174, Carbohydrates: 23 g, Fiber: 6 g, Fat: 7 g, Protein: 7 g

Customizable Granola Bars (Vegetarian & Gluten-Free)

Prep time: 20 minutes

Cook time: 5 minutes

Total time: 25 minutes

Ingredients

1 large cup of pitted dates

¼ cup of honey

½ cup of all-natural almond butter

1 cup roasted unsalted almonds

1 ½ cups of oats (gluten-free for GF eaters)

Optional dark chocolate chips, vanilla extract, etc.

Instructions

1. Add dates to a food processor and process until a dough forms. Set aside.

2. Add the honey and almond butter to a saucepan and heat until melted.

3. Add the almonds, oats, and date dough into a large mixing bowl. Add the almond butter mixture to the bowl and stir well.

4. Pour the mixture into a large pan lined with parchment paper. Flatten with your hands and place the pan in the fridge. Let sit for about 20 minutes, or until firm.

5. Cut into bars or squares and enjoy!

Note: For a vegan option, do not include chocolate chips.

Nutrition Information

(For 1 medium bar)

Calories: 231, Carbohydrates: 34 g, Fiber: 4 g, Fat: 10 g, Protein: 6 g

Apple Peanut Yogurt Dip (Vegetarian & Gluten-Free)

Prep time: 15 minutes

Cook time: 0 minutes

Total time: 15 minutes

Ingredients

1 cup of unsweetened Greek yogurt

⅓ cup of natural peanut butter

2 tablespoons of natural honey

Optional cinnamon or other spices

Instructions

1. Add all ingredients to a bowl and mix well.

2. Add optional cinnamon or other spices.

3. Enjoy with apple slices or on whole-grain bread.

Nutrition Information

(For 4 tablespoons)

Calories: 113, Carbohydrates: 6 g, Fiber: 1 g, Protein: 7 g, Fat: 7 g

Perimenopause Cooking: Key Takeaways

Perimenopause is a difficult pill for many women to swallow. Your body is changing, and oftentimes the onset of these changes feels uncomfortable.

Instead of reaching for over-the-counter medications, focus on fueling your body with intention. Give it the essential vitamins and minerals it needs.

Your doctor may advise you to take supplements or vitamins to help with hormonal changes, so listen to them!

If that isn't the case, starting with a healthy diet can mitigate some of the symptoms of menopause. And, even better, combining these healthy recipes with intermittent fasting amplifies the benefits.

Try this healthy five-day meal plan if you're experiencing the symptoms of perimenopause. You'll be glad you did.

Chapter 7:
Mid-Menopause

"Look at your body and whisper *there is no home like you.* Thank you."

-rupi kaur

We're in the nitty gritty.

Mid-menopause can be pretty uncomfortable; the bright side is that you've already experienced many of the common symptoms! The downside is that your body is changing rapidly.

Many women in mid-menopause feel a bit lost or confused: the worst should be over right?

Change your mindset. Think back to puberty: You likely felt uncomfortable, awkward and a little confused. What was happening? Why? And will it ever end?

It's just like that! You're older, wiser, and better able to cope with what's going on in your body.

Let's talk about what's going on.

What Is Mid-Menopause?

Mid-menopause refers to the period when your body stops producing estrogen and progesterone. If it's been one year since you experienced your last period, you're likely in mid-menopause.

As a generalization, most women enter mid-menopause between the ages of 45 and 55, with an average onset age of 51.

Mid-menopause and perimenopause bring similar symptoms; however, because your body stops producing hormones during mid-menopause, you might notice your symptoms becoming more severe. Most women report hot flashes and vaginal dryness when entering mid-menopause. Some women report sleep disturbances and low bone density, which can lead to injury and fractures.

You might also notice some shifts in mood and sex drive. Some women report these symptoms during perimenopause, but, for many, these symptoms become more prevalent in mid-menopause.

As your moods become irregular, you might lose interest in sex. Your body is no longer producing sex hormones, and you might feel decreased sexual desire. Don't panic just yet!

I'll talk about phytoestrogens in the next step, but dietary habits and planning are key ways to cope with mid-menopause symptoms, including sexual discomfort and low interest.

Give yourself extra time to get aroused and use a water-based lubricant during sexual intercourse. Discuss your concerns with a partner and give yourself ample time to explore your body on your own.

Again, mid-menopause is an unfortunate reality, but with a little tact and planning, you can mitigate some of these symptoms.

The Mid-Menopause Diet

Mid-menopause is the thick of it and paying attention to your diet and nutrition is of high importance. Eating greens, dairy, and whole grains are great ways to keep your body healthy and prepared for everything mid-menopause throws your way.

Dairy Products

Low-fat dairy products, like milk, certain cheeses, and greek yogurt are here to help with all of your mid-menopause symptoms. These foods contain calcium, vitamin D, and potassium, otherwise known as the essential nutrients for bone health and maintenance.

Beyond bone health, low-fat dairy products may improve sleep quality. A recent study showed "that foods high in the amino acid glycine," primary amino acid in milk and cheese products, plays a role in regulating our sleep cycle. (Groves, 2018). The study illustrated a lower incidence of sleep disturbances in those who consumed more low-fat dairy products.

Experts recommend all adults consume about three servings of low-fat dairy per day. This can look like 1 cup of low-fat dairy or fortified soy milk, 2 ounces of cheese, or half a cup of low-fat, plain Greek yogurt.

Try a yogurt parfait for breakfast with a cup of milk and use a little bit of cheese when cooking dinner.

Whole Grains

Whole grains are a common theme in the menopause-mitigating diet; whole grains contain vital nutrients like fiber, niacin, and pantothenic acid.

One study found that participants who consumed three servings of whole grains had a "20-30% lower risk of developing heart disease and diabetes, compared to people who ate mostly refined carbs" (Groves, 2018).

Dietary guidelines dictate that women should aim for sixteen grams of whole grains per day or three servings.

One serving of whole grains looks like any of the following: half a cup of whole grain pasta, 1 slice of whole grain bread, half a cup of brown rice, or half a cup of whole grain hot cereal.

Start your day with whole grain toast and try a nice whole grain pasta and salmon dish for dinner! With a little tact, you can easily hit your whole grain goals.

Phytoestrogens

Phytoestrogens are weak hormones that mimic estrogen in the body and may help minimize menopause symptoms.

Foods like soybeans, chickpeas, grapes, green tea, peanuts, and barley contain phytoestrogen compounds.

Some studies point to higher phytoestrogen consumption and lower incidents of hot flashes in its participants because of their role as a weak estrogen hormone.

Kinda cool, right? Remember, protein, complex carbs, healthy fats, and fruits and veggies are important dietary additions, regardless of age.

The Mid-Menopause Healthy Meal Plan

It's important to note that alcohol, caffeine, sugary beverages, and spicy foods should be eliminated (or decreased) from your diet during mid-menopause. If you need a refresher, look back at Chapter 6.

However, the addition to the "try not to eat" list during mid-menopause is salt. Salt intake is linked to lower bone density in women during menopause.

A sodium intake higher than 2 grams daily has been linked to a 28% higher risk of low bone density in women between the ages of 50 and 60. Lowering your salt intake decreases bloating and brain fog while improving bone density and cardiovascular function.

In the next section, I'll introduce a five-day meal plan for women undergoing mid-menopause. Each of these recipes is chock full of mid-menopause healthy ingredients, like whole grains, phytoestrogens, and low-fat dairy products to get you going on your journey.

You got this!

Breakfast

Homemade Healthy Granola (Vegan & Gluten-Free)

Prep time: 10 minutes

Cook time: 20 minutes

Total time: 30 minutes

Ingredients

4 cups rolled oats

1 ½ cups raw pecans

1 teaspoon salt

½ teaspoon cinnamon

½ cup coconut oil

½ cup honey

1 teaspoon vanilla extract

⅔ cup dried cranberries or desired fruit

Instructions

1. Preheat your oven to 350 degrees F.

2. Combine oats, pecans, salt, and cinnamon in a large mixing bowl and stir.

3. Add the oil, honey, and vanilla and mix until well-coated.

4. Spread the granola onto a large baking sheet lined with parchment. Ensure the layer is nice and even.

5. Bake in the oven for about 20 minutes.

6. Let the granola cool for an hour, and top it with optional chocolate chips!

Nutrition Information

(For a ½ cup serving without toppings)

Amount Per Serving

Calories: 234, Carbohydrates: 28 g, Fiber: 3 g, Protein: 4 g, Fat: 12 g

Blueberry & Avocado Smoothie (Vegan & Gluten-Free)

Prep time: 10 minutes

Cook time: 0 minutes

Total time: 10 minutes

Ingredients

½ cup unsweetened almond milk (vanilla is my favorite)

1 cup spinach

1 medium pre-peeled banana

½ peeled and pre-pitted avocado

2 cups frozen blueberries

1 tablespoon ground flaxseed

1 tablespoon unsweetened almond butter

½ teaspoon ground cinnamon

Instructions

1. Add all the ingredients to your blender or food processor.

2. Blend everything until nice and smooth.

3. Enjoy!

Nutrition Information

(For one serving, the recipe makes two)

Calories: 283, Carbohydrates: 42 g, Fiber: 11 g, Protein: 6 g, Fat: 13 g

Easy Banana Breakfast Bowl (Vegan & Gluten-Free)

Prep time: 20 minutes

Cook time: 10 minutes

Total time: 30 minutes

Ingredients

2 pre-peeled bananas

¾ cup grapes

⅔ cup shelled walnuts

1 tablespoon coconut oil

1 tablespoon honey

½ teaspoon cinnamon

Instructions

1. Slice the bananas into medium slices and cut the grapes in half. Preheat a large skillet over medium-high heat and add the coconut oil. Place the banana slices on the pan and sauté for about 3 minutes. Flip, then sauté the other side. Place the banana in individual bowls.

2. Use the same pan and add the nuts, grapes, honey, and cinnamon and sauté for 3 minutes.

3. Add the nut mixture to the bowls and enjoy!

Nutrition Information

(If making 4 servings)

Calories: 243, Carbohydrates: 24 g, Fiber: 3 g, Protein: 4 g, Fat: 17 g

Healthy Blueberry Muffins (Vegan)

Prep time: 20 minutes

Cook time: 20 minutes

Total time: 40 minutes

Ingredients

1 ½ cups white whole wheat flour and one extra tablespoon

¾ cup rolled oats

½ cup light brown sugar

1 tablespoon baking powder

½ teaspoon cinnamon

½ teaspoon salt

1 cup almond milk

¼ cup melted coconut oil

2 large eggs

2 teaspoons vanilla extract

1 cup frozen blueberries

Instructions

1. Preheat your oven to 400 degrees F and coat a muffin tray with cooking spray.

2. Combine the 1 ½ cups of flour, oats, baking powder, salt, sugar, and cinnamon, and stir well.

3. For the wet ingredients, whisk eggs, vanilla, milk, and butter together in a separate bowl.

4. Add a bit of the wet ingredients to the dry ingredients and stir. Continue until all of the wet ingredients are well combined.

5. Coat the blueberries with the extra flour and add them to the batter.

6. Add the batter to the muffin tin and bake for about 20 minutes.

7. Let them cool and enjoy!

Nutrition Information

(For 1 muffin)

Calories: 165, Carbohydrates: 26 g, Fiber: 2 g, Protein: 4 g, Fat: 5 g

Autumn Cranberry Pumpkin Loaf (Vegetarian & Gluten-Free)

Prep time: 30 minutes

Cook time: 70 minutes

Total time: 1 hour and 40 minutes

Ingredients

1½ cups halved raw walnuts

1 cup raw pumpkin seeds

2¾ cups rolled oats

1 cup dried cranberries

¾ cup mixed flaxseeds and chia seeds

⅓ cup psyllium husks

Salt to taste

¾ teaspoon cinnamon

½ teaspoon nutmeg

1 can of unsweetened pumpkin puree

1 cup water

¼ cup natural maple syrup

¼ cup melted coconut oil

Instructions

1. Preheat your oven to 325 degrees F.

2. Place walnuts and seeds on a lined baking sheet and bake for about 10 minutes. They should appear nice and golden.

3. Combine oats, seeds, husks, salt, cranberries, cinnamon, and nutmeg in a medium mixing bowl and stir. Then add the walnuts and seeds.

4. Add pumpkin, about 1 cup of water, syrup, and melted coconut oil to the bowl and wait until a nice dough forms.

5. Use parchment paper to line a large loaf pan and press down. Try to round the loaf on top a bit. Cover with plastic wrap and let it sit at room temperature for about three hours.

6. Raise the oven temperature to 400 degrees F and bake to loaf for about an hour and ten minutes. It will look bronzy on top when it's done.

7. Let it cool and enjoy!

Nutrition Information

(For 1 small slice)

Calories: 534, Carbohydrates: 31 g, Fiber: 20 g, Protein: 17 g, Fat: 43 g

Lunch

Fall Squash Soup (Vegan & Gluten-Free)

Prep time: 15 minutes

Cook time: 25 minutes

Total time: 40 minutes

Ingredients

½ tablespoon olive oil

2 minced garlic cloves

1 diced white onion

1 butternut squash pre-diced into small cubes

32 ounces vegetable broth (if you're not following a vegan recipe, chicken broth is okay)

Salt to taste

Instructions

1. Heat the oil in a large pot over medium-low heat. Next, add the onion and garlic; cook until fragrant, or for about 6 minutes.

2. Add the squash and broth to the pot and bring to a nice boil. Once boiling, reduce heat to low and cover for about 20 minutes.

3. Wait until the mixture has cooled before adding it to a blender or food processor. Process until smooth and add a pinch of salt.

4. Serve in 1-cup portions.

Nutrition Information

Calories: 135, Carbohydrates: 24 g, Fiber: 3 g, Protein: 1 g, Fat: 4 g

Healthy Orzo Salad (Pescatarian)

Prep time: 20 minutes

Cook time: 15 minutes

Total time: 35 minutes

Ingredients

½ chopped red onion

2 tablespoons sherry vinegar

1 ¼ cup green beans, cut into bite-sized pieces

¾ cup orzo

1 tablespoon extra-virgin olive oil

1 small can of pre-drained tuna

3 chopped roasted red peppers

12 halved black olives

a handful of dill, chopped

Salt and pepper to taste

Instructions

1. Combine onions and sherry vinegar in a small mixing bowl and lightly season with salt and pepper.

2. Bring a large pot of water to a boil and salt lightly. Cook the green beans for about 3-5 minutes and remove them from the water.

3. Add the orzo to the same pot and cook according to the directions. Then, rise the orzo in water and set it aside.

4. Add the remaining ingredients to the onion mixture and stir well.

Note: Topping with thinly sliced cucumbers makes for a delicious addition to the salad!

Nutrition Information

Calories: 298, Carbohydrates: 27 g, Fiber: 5 g, Protein: 19 g, Fat: 12 g

Cauliflower Lentil Bowl (Vegan & Gluten-Free)

Prep time: 15 minutes

Cook time: 40 minutes

Total time: 55 minutes

Ingredients

¾ cup lentils

6 ounces cauliflower florets

1 tablespoon curry powder

2 small sweet peppers

4 ounces of red grapes

1 ripe avocado

2 tablespoon balsamic vinaigrette

4 ounces Arcadian greens

Salt and pepper to taste

1 teaspoon extra-virgin olive oil

Instructions

1. Preheat your oven to 425 degrees F.

2. Next, rinse the lentils and add them to a small saucepan with about 2 cups of water. Bring the lentils to a boil and then reduce the heat to medium-low. Simmer for about 25 minutes. The lentils are done when the water is fully absorbed. Season with salt and pepper.

3. Add the olive oil to a baking sheet with the cauliflower and season with curry powder and salt and pepper. Roast in the preheated oven for about 10 minutes.

4. Slice the small peppers and cut the grapes into halves. Remove the pit and flesh from the avocado and slice the flesh into small pieces.

5. Combine the vinaigrette and salt into a small bowl and whisk together.

6. Add the greens into two large serving bowls and add a small tablespoon of the vinaigrette.

7. Finally, add the remaining ingredients and mix just a bit!

Nutrition Information

Calories: 530, Carbohydrates: 73 g, Fiber: 27 g, Protein: 24 g, Fat: 18 g

Baked Falafel (Vegan & Gluten-Free)

Prep time: 15 minutes

Cook time: 35 minutes

Total time: 45 minutes

Ingredients

1 15 oz can of pre-drained chickpeas

½ cup diced white onion

1 cup parsley

1 cup cilantro

Salt and pepper to taste

1 teaspoon coriander

1 teaspoon garlic powder

2 teaspoons baking powder

2 teaspoons cumin

2 tablespoons flaxseed

1 tablespoon extra-virgin olive oil

Instructions

1. Preheat your oven to 400 degrees F.

2. In a food processor, add the onions, chickpeas, parsley, and cilantro. Process until combined. Add the salt, pepper, and remaining ingredients (not the olive oil) to the processor and combine well. The mixture should look like dough.

3. Grease a large baking sheet with olive oil.

4. Roll the falafel dough into small balls and flatten them with a drinking glass. Space them on the baking sheet and cook for about 20 minutes. Flip the falafel after 20 minutes and cook for an additional 15 minutes.

5. Let cool and serve with whole grain pita bread.

Nutrition Information

(For 1 falafel)

Calories: 38, Carbohydrates: 5 g, Fiber: 1 g, Protein: 1 g, Fat: 1 g

Summer Rolls (Vegan)

Prep time: 35 minutes

Cook time: 0 minutes

Total time: 35 minutes

Ingredients

1 tablespoons ginger

1 teaspoon chili powder

4 tablespoons rice vinegar

2 tablespoons low-sodium soy sauce

1 tablespoon sesame oil

Lime juice

2 tablespoons agave syrup

1 teaspoon sesame seeds

3 large carrots

1 medium cucumber

1 cup red cabbage

1 medium mango

3 radishes

1 ripe avocado

7 sheets of rice paper

Instructions

1. Chop the ginger and combine it with rice vinegar, soy sauce, a bit of water, agave, lime juice, oil, and sesame seeds in a large bowl.
2. Slice carrots, cabbage, and cucumber into small pieces. Next, slice mango, avocado meat, and radish.
3. Add water to a large mixing bowl and wet the rice paper with the water. Lay the rice paper on a flat surface.
4. Assemble the wraps and make sure to seal the slides of the rice wrap.
5. Enjoy!

Nutrition Information

(For 1 wrap)

Calories: 177, Carbohydrates: 26 g, Fiber: 5 g, Protein: 3 g, Fat: 6 g

Dinner

Chicken Satay

Prep time: 20 minutes

Cook time: 15 minutes

Total time: 35 minutes

Ingredients
Satay
1½ lb. pre-cubed Chicken Breast
2 tablespoons extra-virgin olive oil
1 tablespoon curry powder
1 teaspoon garlic salt
1 tablespoon honey
2 teaspoons of curry paste
Salt and pepper to taste
A small handful of roasted peanuts
Peanut Sauce
3 tablespoons lemon juice
2 tablespoons low-sodium soy sauce
⅓ cup of natural smooth peanut butter
1 tablespoon apple cider vinegar
1 tablespoon sriracha
Some water to thin the ingredients

Instructions

1. Combine chicken, curry powder, oil, garlic salt, honey, paste, and salt and pepper in a large mixing bowl. Let sit for about 15 minutes.

2. Place the marinated chicken bites onto skewers. Heat a grill pan to medium heat and cook for a few minutes on each side. This should take about 5 minutes total.

3. Make your sauce. Whisk all the ingredients together in a small bowl and add water if needed.

4. Drizzle the sauce over the skewers and top with chopped peanuts.

Notes: Serve over brown rice for a well-rounded meal!

Nutrition Information

(For 2 skewers)

Calories: 415, Carbohydrates: 12 g, Fiber: 2 g, Protein: 42 g, Fat: 23 g

Salmon Foil Package (Pescatarian & Gluten-Free)

Prep time: 15 minutes

Cook time: 20 minutes

Total time: 35 minutes

Ingredients

4 salmon fillets with skin removed

Salt and pepper to taste

1 pound of pre-trimmed asparagus

1 thinly sliced lemon

½ cup room temperature unsalted butter (trust me!)

2 teaspoons of Italian seasoning of your choice

3 teaspoons of minced garlic

Lemon juice

Instructions

1. Preheat the oven to 100 degrees F.

2. Place salmon filets and some of the asparagus (about a quarter) on a large piece of foil and season with salt and pepper. Do the same with each filet, using separate pieces of foil. Place the lemon slices under the filets.

3. Mix butter and seasonings in a mixing bowl until combined. Add the butter in equal amounts to each of the foil packages.

4. Fold the packages and make sure to seal the edges. Bake for about 20 minutes or until the salmon is no longer bright pink.

5. Drizzle lemon juice on each of the opened packages before serving.

Note: Serve over brown rice!

Nutrition Information

(For 1 package)

Calories: 286, Carbohydrates: 7 g, Fiber: 2 g, Protein: 37 g, Fat: 12 g

Healthy Spaghetti and Meatballs (Gluten-Free)

Prep time: 15 minutes

Cook time: About 20 minutes

Total time: 35 minutes

Ingredients

Zoodles

4 medium spiralized Zucchini

2 cups low-sodium Marinara Sauce

2 tablespoons grated romano or parmesan cheese

Meatballs

1 ½ lbs. lean ground turkey

¼ cup grated parmesan cheese

1 room temperature egg

1 tablespoon Italian seasoning

Salt and pepper to taste

Instructions

1. Preheat your oven to 400 degrees F. Spray a large baking sheet with nonstick spray.

2. Combine all the meatball ingredients in a large bowl and stir well. Create small meatballs and add them to the baking sheet. Cook for about 16 minutes or until fully cooked.

3. Divide the zoodles into 4 servings and place them in serving bowls. Top with the marinara sauce and stir to coat. Finally, add the meatballs and cheese! Enjoy.

Nutrition Information

(For 1 bowl or ¼ serving)

Calories: 311, Carbohydrates: 14 g, Fiber: 4 g, Protein: 49 g, Fat: 7 g

Sweet Barbeque Chicken (Gluten-Free)

Prep time: 35 minutes

Cook time: 15 minutes

Total time: 50 minutes

Ingredients

1 ⅓ lb. skinless chicken breast

½ cup low-sugar barbecue sauce

¼ cup of pineapple juice

2 tablespoons of low-sodium soy sauce

1 garlic clove, pre-minced

1 teaspoon pre-minded ginger

2 cups of pineapple cut into slices

Instructions

1. Combine pineapple juice, barbecue sauce, soy sauce garlic, and ginger in a large bowl or gallon-size plastic bag. Let sit for over 30 minutes.

2. Pat the chicken dry and add to a preheated grill, cooking for about 5 minutes. Spray the pineapple slices with nonstick cooking spray and grill them for 5 minutes as well.

3. Add the excess marinade to a small saucepan and let cook for about 5 minutes or until slightly thickened.

4. Drizzle the marinade over the chicken and serve over brown rice!

Nutrition Information

(For 6 ounces of chicken and 2 slices of pineapple)

Calories: 270, Carbohydrates: 25 g, Fiber: 2 g, Protein: 33 g, Fat: 2 g

Shrimp & Pasta Dinner Salad (Pescatarian)

Prep time: 15 minutes

Cook time: 10 minutes

Total time: 25 minutes

Ingredients

Shrimp & Pasta

8 ounces uncooked whole wheat macaroni

1 lb. cooked shrimp, peeled and deveined

2 stalks of celery, diced

1 diced red bell pepper

1 cup thawed pre-frozen peas

½ cup chopped green onions

2 tablespoons chopped dill

Dressing

⅔ cup plain greek yogurt

Lemon juice

2 teaspoons natural honey

1 teaspoon of white vinegar

½ teaspoon of Dijon mustard

Salt and pepper to taste

Instructions

1. Cook the pasta according to package instructions and drain in a colander.

2. Whisk the dressing ingredients together in a small mixing bowl.

3. Combine the remaining pasta and shrimp ingredients (shrimp, celery, pepper, onion, peas, dill) in a large serving bowl and add the pasta. Stir well to thoroughly combine.

4. Add the dressing. Eat up!

Note: The recipe can be made gluten-free with gluten-free pasta!

Nutrition Information

(For ⅛ of the recipe)

Calories: 194, Carbohydrates: 28 g, Fiber: 1 g, Protein: 19 g, Fat: 1 g

Snacks

Chia Seed Pudding (Vegan & Gluten-Free)

Prep time: 10 minutes

Cook time: 0 minutes

Total time: About 6 hours (for the pudding to thicken)

Ingredients

¾ cup unsweetened almond milk

1 tablespoon of natural honey

1 teaspoon vanilla extract

3 tablespoons of chia seeds

Optional halved raspberries for topping

Instructions

1. Add all ingredients to a small mason jar and stir with a small spoon to prevent any lumps from forming.

2. Refrigerate for about 6 hours or overnight.

3. Remove from the fridge and stir the pudding before adding your optional toppings!

Nutrition Information

Calories: 265, Carbohydrates: 33 g, Fiber: 13 g , Protein: 7 g , Fat: 13 g

A Non-Millennial's Avocado Toast (Can Be Made Vegan)

Prep time: 5 minutes

Cook time: About 5 minutes

Total time: 10 minutes

Ingredients

1 avocado

2 tablespoons cilantro

Lime juice

Salt and pepper to taste

2 slices of whole grain bread

Optional 2 fried eggs

Instructions

1. Toast the whole grain bread for three minutes in your toaster.

2. Combine avocado, cilantro, salt and pepper, and lime juice in a small mixing bowl.

3. Spread the avocado mixture on top of the toast.

4. Add a fried egg for an extra protein punch if you'd like and enjoy!

Nutrition Facts (with the egg included)

(Serves 2)

Calories: 332, Carbohydrates: 24 g, Fiber: 10 g, Protein: 12 g, Fat: 23 g

Homemade Guacamole (Vegan & Gluten-Free)

Prep time: 15 minutes

Cook time: 0 minutes

Total time: 15 minutes

Ingredients

2 ripe avocados, peeled

2 cloves of garlic, minced

Lime juice

Salt to taste

¼ cup diced red onion

Instructions

1. Scoop the meat out of the avocado and set it aside. Add the avocado meat to a large mixing bowl and add the minced garlic. Stir to combine.

2. Add the lime juice, salt, and red onion. Stir well.

3. Enjoy!

Note: Use veggies or whole-grain pita chips to scoop guacamole.

Nutrition Information

(For ¼ of the recipe)

Calories: 168, Carbohydrates: 11 g, Fiber: 7 g, Protein: 2 g, Fat: 15 g

Dark Chocolate-Covered Almonds (Vegetarian & Gluten-Free)

Prep time: 15 minutes

Cook time: 0 minutes

Cool time: 3 hours

Total time: 3 hours and 15 minutes

Ingredients

1 ½ cups raw unsalted almonds

7 oz dark chocolate (the higher the % of the chocolate, the better)

Optional sea salt

Instructions

1. Chop up the chocolate and add to a microwave-safe bowl. Microwave for about 20 seconds, then stir. You may need to repeat this step a few times until all the chocolate is melted.

2. Add all of the almonds to the bowl of chocolate and use a fork to coat each almond.

3. Place each almond on a parchment paper lined sheet pan and place in the refrigerator to dry for about three hours.

4. Enjoy!

Note: This is a great topping for fruit, trail mix, or even low-fat ice cream!

Nutrition Information

(Recipe makes 15 servings; nutrition information is for 1 serving)

Calories: 161, Carbohydrates: 9 g, Fiber: 3 g, Protein: 4 g, Fat: 13 g

Food Is The Cure: Mid-Menopause Diet

Suffering from hot flashes?

Try homemade hummus.

Sleep disturbances?

Reach for the cottage cheese celery sticks.

Is it feeling a little uncomfy down there?

It's time for a glass of green tea.

Mid-menopause stinks; no one's disputing that. Consider what I've asked you to do throughout this book: You've been asked to consider alternative ways to combat health issues and bodily changes.

Instead of reaching for a Tums, consider what you ate to trigger your discomfort. You know the drill. Intermittent fasting, coupled with a healthy, nutrient-rich diet, is a great way to combat some of the mental and physical symptoms of menopause.

It's about what you eat when you eat, and what you think about while doing it.

Chapter 8:
Post-Menopause

"Beauty begins the moment you decide to be yourself."

– Coco Chanel

It's not the end quite yet, my friend. That's the tricky thing about menopause: There's no definitive end date. Your body won't simply 'go back' to how it was before: It's a tough pill to swallow.

It's natural. It's human. But it's a little uncomfortable.

There are some key things to watch out for when you're in post-menopause. This Chapter will showcase the symptoms, signs, and ins and outs of post-menopause. I'll also provide you with some recipes to help you cope with these symptoms.

You're not alone.

What Is Post-Menopause?

On a basic level, the term 'post-menopause' refers to the time after mid-menopause. Post-menopause doesn't really end per se; your body might get used to its new hormone levels, but there isn't a definitive endpoint. Some women report fewer or more mild menopause symptoms, and some report no symptoms at all. For the most part, one can expect a few changes, but there's nothing to be afraid of.

Women in post-menopause report some of the following symptoms:

- Hot flashes and night sweats
- Depression and mood changes
- Discomfort during intercourse
- Insomnia or irregular sleep patterns
- Dry skin or acne
- Weight gain
- Urinary incontinence

But why do some of these symptoms arise? What's going on?

Keep reading.

Concerns During Post-Menopause

Many women in post-menopause become more sedentary due to fatigue and irregular sleep patterns. Sedentary behavior can trigger increases in cholesterol and blood pressure levels, and, over time, high blood pressure and high cholesterol contribute to the development of heart disease.

Moving more and eating a healthy diet can keep these factors at bay.

Estrogen plays a pivotal role in bone maintenance so when your body stops producing it, it's likely you'll begin to lose bone density. You can lose up to 2% of your bone density per year during post-menopause.

Low bone density can cause osteoporosis, leading to broken bones and slow recovery time. Exercising and eating a healthy diet (I'll go into diet more later in the chapter) can help you prevent osteoporosis and maintain your bone density!

You'll likely experience vaginal dryness during the earlier stages of menopause, but, unfortunately, vaginal dryness is the chief complaint among post-menopausal women.

When your body produces less estrogen, your vaginal walls become thinner (called vaginal atrophy), causing vaginal dryness. Use a water-based lubricant during sexual intercourse to reduce pain and discomfort.

You might also experience a lack of bladder control; if this is the case, talk to your doctor.

What to Eat

A healthy diet (while intermittent fasting) is a theme throughout every stage of menopause. However, there are a few dietary tweaks to be made between each stage. Let's talk about some dietary considerations for women in post-menopause!

Vitamin C Rich Foods

Vitamin C is a cool vitamin: It plays a role in both bone maintenance and density and antiaging. Vitamin C is an antioxidant and aids in the reduction of potentially harmful cells that could cause heart disease or cancer in the body.

When estrogen levels decrease (as they do in post-menopause) our bodies and cells become more susceptible to oxidative stress and damage. In short, vitamin C is pretty important.

We went into vitamin C in detail in the perimenopause chapter as well, so review chapter 6 if you need a refresher. Consume plenty of bell peppers, citrus fruits, broccoli, cauliflower, and tomatoes to boost your ability to fight infection, age gracefully, and maintain bone density.

Dietary Phytoestrogens

We discussed phytoestrogens in the previous chapter, but their importance is certainly worth reiterating.

Dietary phytoestrogens are foods that contain compounds similar to the hormone estrogen. Essentially, dietary phytoestrogens mimic estrogen in the body which can mitigate some of the symptoms of post-menopause.

Foods like soybeans or soymilk, flaxseeds, and oats contain phytoestrogens.

Unsaturated Fats

Because post-menopause can trigger high blood pressure and high cholesterol, it's our job to counteract those symptoms with heart-healthy foods.

Unsaturated fats are liquid at room temperature; they can lower your cholesterol and reduce unwanted inflammation.

Foods like avocado, olive oil, almonds, and pumpkin seeds all contain unsaturated, heart-healthy fats.

Calcium

It's no secret that calcium supports strong bones. Because decreased bone density is often a symptom of post-menopause, we must maintain healthy calcium levels to keep our bones healthy and ready to move!

I went into more detail about calcium in the perimenopause chapter, so I'll keep it short: try eating plenty of salmon, low-fat dairy products, chia seeds, beans, and almonds!

Vitamin D

Vitamin D plays a strong role in calcium absorption, ultimately aiding your bone health. On top of that vitamin D can help maintain regular sleep patterns.

Vitamin D is a fat-soluble vitamin; you can obtain vitamin D from the sun, but most people can make vitamin D on their own too! That isn't to say you shouldn't ingest vitamin D on a daily basis. It's a necessity.

Certain studies show that "vitamin D can reduce cancer cell growth, help control infections and reduce inflammation" (*Vitamin D*, 2021). Most of your body's organs have external vitamin D receptors; we're pre-programmed to need it.

Many of the body's organs and tissues have receptors for vitamin D, which suggest important roles beyond bone health, and scientists are actively investigating other possible functions.

Studies regarding vitamin D are relatively limited; it would be unethical to knowingly deprive someone of a nutrient they need! However, observational studies are readily available and show that adequate vitamin D consumption plays a role in bone health, certain types of cancers, depression, anxiety, weight gain, heart disease, and type 2 diabetes.

Dietary guidelines for vitamin D vary a bit, but in general, all American adults should consume about 15 micrograms (mcg) of vitamin D daily, regardless of the time they spend outside.

It's not too hard to hit this goal; you got this! Three ounces of salmon contains just over fourteen mcg of vitamin D, and three ounces of trout or rainbow fish offers sixteen. Half a cup of mushrooms equates to about 9 mcg, a cup of soy milk provides 3 more, and an egg contains one mcg of vitamin D. Other drinks like vitamin D-fortified milk or orange juice pack another vitamin D-filled punch.

For example, if you eat two eggs with a cup of soy milk for breakfast and three ounces of salmon for dinner, you're well past your vitamin D goal for the day.

Five-Day Post-Menopause Food Plan

This chapter, just like the last two, will introduce five days of meal and snack recipes to get you started on your post-menopausal health journey. These recipes can be tailored and changed to fit your intermittent fasting plan; if you're engaging in a 16:8 model, try one lunch and one dinner recipe! You choose how and when you eat.

Each of these recipes contains great post-menopause-healthy ingredients, including vitamin D, calcium, and phytoestrogens.

Along that line, feel free to alter these recipes as you'd like. If you're not an almond fan, try walnuts or peanuts!

You're more likely to stick with it if you're staying true to yourself and your needs!

Breakfast

Breakfast Chocolate Oatmeal (Vegan & Gluten-Free)

Prep time: 5 minutes

Cook time: 10 minutes

Total time: 15 minutes

Ingredients

1 heaping cup of rolled oats

1 cup of unsweetened almond milk

3 tablespoons of unsweetened cocoa powder

2 tablespoons of natural maple syrup

½ teaspoons vanilla extract

½ teaspoon of cinnamon

Pinch of salt

Optional: dark chocolate chips, sliced almonds, sliced strawberries, etc

Instructions

1. Add all of the ingredients to a medium saucepan. Stir well and cook over medium heat until the mixture is creamy. Continue to stir.

2. Pour into 2 bowls and enjoy!

Nutrition Information

Calories: 215, Carbohydrates: 39 g, Fiber: 8 g, Protein: 7 g, Fat: 0.5 g

Huevos Rancheros (Vegetarian & Gluten-Free)

Prep time: 15 minutes

Cook time: 30 minutes

Total time: 45 minutes

Ingredients

1 small white pre-chopped onion

½ teaspoon of ground cumin

½ teaspoon of ground paprika

2 ¼ cups of canned black beans

1 chopped Roma tomato

4 small corn tortillas

1 ripe avocado

½ cup of seeds of your choosing

2 large eggs

½ tablespoon of melted coconut oil

Salt and pepper to taste

Instructions

1. Add the melted coconut oil to a large saucepan and add ¾ of the chopped onion. Caramelize them slightly, stirring continuously.
2. Add cumin, paprika, seeds, salt, and pepper, and cook for another minute. Continue to stir, then add the beans and some water.
3. Let cook for about 20-25 minutes and continue to stir.
4. Use the remaining ¼ of chopped onion, tomato, and a bit more salt to make the salsa. Stir well in a small mixing bowl and set aside.
5. Scramble the eggs in a separate pan and then set them aside. Warm the tortillas in the same pan and set them aside.
6. Remove the meat from the avocado and mix it with the seeds in a small mixing bowl.
7. The recipe serves four, so to assemble, place 2 tortillas each on plates and add the bean mixture. Spread the salsa on top and add the egg. Finally, spread the avocado over the egg and enjoy!

Nutrition Information

Calories: 619, Carbohydrates: 94 g, Fiber: 24 g, Protein: 31 g, Fat: 15 g

PB & J Chia Seed Pudding (Gluten-Free & Vegan)

Prep time: 20 minutes

Cook time: 1 hour (varies)

Total time: 1 hour and 20 minutes

Ingredients

1 cup of frozen blueberries

1 tablespoon of pulp-free, unsweetened orange juice

1 tablespoon and ⅓ cup of chia seeds

1 ½ cups of unsweetened almond milk

Maple syrup to taste

3 tablespoons of natural almond butter

Instructions

1. Combine blueberries and orange juice in a small saucepan and cook over medium heat until the mixture just begins to bubble. Lower the heat slightly and cook for another few minutes (2-3). Then stir in the tablespoon of chia seeds after removing the pan from heat.

2. Add the compote in even amounts to three mason jars or small ramekins and let the compote sit in the refrigerator to cool down.

3. Combine syrup, almond milk, and almond butter in a blender and blend well to fully combine. Next, add the rest of the chia seeds and continue to blend.

4. Add the blender mixture to a small bowl and place in the fridge to chill a bit, or for about 10 minutes.

5. Add the chia seed blender mixture to the ramekins and chill for another few hours before serving!

Nutrition Information

(For ⅓ of the recipe)

Calories: 211, Carbohydrates: 19 g, Fiber: 6 g, Protein: 6 g, Fat: 13 g

Oatmeal Pancakes (Vegetarian & Gluten-Free)

Prep time: 15 minutes

Cook time: 10 minutes

Total time: 25 minutes

Ingredients

2 medium bananas

2 large eggs

½ cup of unsweetened almond milk

1 teaspoon of vanilla extract

1 ½ cups of rolled oats

2 teaspoons of baking powder

½ teaspoon ground cinnamon

Coconut oil for cooking

Instructions

1. Blend all of the ingredients in a blender or food processor until nice and batter-like. Let it sit for a few minutes to emulsify.

2. Add coconut oil to a large skillet and let it warm over medium heat.

3. Add about 1/9th of the batter to the skillet and cook until both sides of the pancake are browned.

4. Repeat with remaining batter and serve warm!

Note: You can add natural maple syrup to the top for a yummy breakfast treat!

Nutrition Information

(For ⅓ of the recipe)

Calories: 311, Carbohydrates: 52 g, Fiber: 7 g, Protein: 12 g, Fat: 7 g

Gluten-Free Banana Bread (Vegetarian & Gluten-Free)

Prep time: 15 minutes

Cook time: 40 minutes

Total time: 55 minutes

Ingredients

2 cups of almond flour

1 teaspoon of baking soda

¾ teaspoon of baking powder

Salt to taste

Optional mini dark-chocolate chips

1 ½ mashed banana

½ cup greek yogurt

½ cup of honey

⅓ cup of unsweetened almond milk

2 teaspoons of vanilla extract

Instructions

1. Line a loaf pan with parchment paper and preheat your oven to 350 degrees F.

2. Combine flour, baking soda and extract, and salt, in a medium mixing bowl. Stir well.

3. Stir together the banana, yogurt, honey, almond milk, and vanilla in a separate bowl until well combined

4. Slowly add the wet ingredients to the dry ones and stir well. The mixture should look like a nice batter.

5. Add the batter to the loaf pan and add desired chocolate chips to the top.

6. Bake for 35-45 minutes. Use a toothpick to test when it's done.

7. Let the bread cool and enjoy warm!

Nutrition Information

(For ⅛ of the recipe)

Calories: 211, Carbohydrates: 29 g, Fiber: 1 g, Protein: 13 g, Fat: 5 g

Lunch

Caesar Salad Wrap
Prep time: 30 minutes
Cook time: 15 minutes
Total time: 45 minutes

Ingredients
1 ½ pounds of chicken breast
1 teaspoon of Italian seasoning
Salt and pepper to taste
Pinch of onion powder and garlic powder
1 ½ tablespoons of extra-virgin olive oil
Lemon juice
⅔ cup of plain, unsweetened greek yogurt
2 teaspoons of Worcestershire sauce
1 teaspoon of dijon mustard
1 clove of garlic
4 large whole-wheat tortillas
1 large head of lettuce, pre-chopped
1 Roma tomato
1 avocado, meat removed
⅓ cup of low-fat mozzarella cheese

Instructions
1. Whisk together the yogurt, sauce, mustard, and garlic in a small mixing bowl and refrigerate for a few minutes.
2. Tenderize the chicken.
3. Preheat your oven to 425 degrees F.
4. Combine the seasonings (salt, Italian seasoning, pepper, onion and garlic powder, oil, and lemon juice) in another bowl and rub over the chicken until evenly coated.
5. Place the chicken on a large baking sheet and cook for about 10-12 minutes. Check to ensure it's done.
6. Add the lettuce, sliced avocado meat, and chopped Roma tomato to a bowl. Give it one stir.
7. Add some of the lettuce mixtures to a tortilla and do the same with each tortilla. Make sure to keep amounts as equal as possible. Add the chicken to each tortilla before adding cheese. Lastly, drizzle the dressing over the "burritos" and enjoy!

Nutrition Information
(For 1 burrito)
Calories: 463, Carbohydrates: 37 g Fiber: 4 g, Protein: 50 g, Fat: 13 g

Tofu Scramble (Vegan & Gluten-Free)

Prep time: 20 minutes

Cook time: 10 minutes

Total time: about 30 minutes

Ingredients

1 tablespoon of extra-virgin olive oil

A 16-ounce block of tofu

2 tablespoons of nutritional yeast

Salt to taste

¼ teaspoon turmeric

A pinch of garlic powder

2 tablespoons of unsweetened almond milk

Instructions

1. Add the olive oil to a large pan and heat over medium. Add the tofu to the pan and mash until it crumbles a bit. Cook for about 4-5 minutes and make sure to stir continuously.

2. Add everything but the milk to the pan and continue to cook for another 5 minutes.

3. Add the almond milk and mix well.

4. Remove from heat and enjoy!

Note: Kale makes a great addition to the recipe should you so choose!

Nutrition Information

(For ½ of the recipe)

Calories: 288, Carbohydrates: 9 g, Fiber: 4 g, Protein: 24 g, Fat: 18 g

Salmon Salad (Pescatarian & Gluten-Free)

Prep time: 15 minutes

Cook time: 10-15 minutes

Total time: 30 minutes

Ingredients

8 ounces of salmon (filet)

3 cups of chopped cucumber

1 ½ of red bell pepper, pre-chopped

¾ cup of chopped red onion

1 medium avocado, pre-chopped and meat removed

4 cups of chopped spinach or lettuce

2 tablespoons of lemon juice

3 tablespoons of extra-virgin olive oil

Salt and pepper to taste

Instructions

1. Cook the salmon on a parchment paper-lined baking sheet in a 400-degree F oven. Bake for about 10-12 minutes or until flakey. Remove and let cool.

2. Add the cooled salmon, cucumber, pepper, onion, lettuce, and avocado to a large mixing bowl to combine.

3. Whisk together the lemon juice, olive oil, and salt and pepper in a small bowl and add to the salad.

4. Enjoy!

Nutrition Information

(For ¼ of the recipe)

Calories: 296, Carbohydrates: 15 g, Fiber: 6 g, Protein: 15 g, Fat: 21 g

Mackerel Pate (Pescatarian & Gluten-Free)

Prep time: 20 minutes

Cook time: 0 minutes

Total time: 20 minutes

Ingredients

4 pre-cooked mackerel filets

2 teaspoons horseradish sauce

2 teaspoons of Dijon mustard

Salt and pepper to taste

2 tablespoons of crème fraiche

Lemon juice

2 tablespoons of coconut oil

Instructions

1. Remove the bones and skin from the pre-cooked mackerel.

2. Add the mackerel, mustard, horseradish, lemon juice, salt and pepper, and crème fraiche to a blender or food processor and blend until it forms a ball. Add the coconut oil and keep blending.

3. Serve on whole wheat bread.

Nutrition Information

(For ¼ or recipe)

Calories: 316, Carbohydrates: 1 g, Fiber: 0 g, Protein: 23 g, Fat: 24 g

Hearty Stuffed Peppers (Gluten-Free)

Prep time: 15 minutes

Cook time: 40-45 minutes

Total time: 55 minutes to 1 hour

Ingredients

4 red bell peppers

2 teaspoons extra-virgin olive oil

1 pound of lean ground chicken

2 teaspoons of Italian seasoning

Salt and pepper to taste

15-ounce can of diced tomatoes

1 ½ cups of pre-cooked brown rice

1 cup of shredded low-fat Mozzarella cheese

½ cup of shredded Parmesan cheese

Basil

Instructions

1. Line a baking sheet with parchment paper and preheat your oven to 375 degrees F.

2. Cut each pepper in half and remove the seeds. Add them to the baking dish.

3. Add chicken, olive oil, and seasonings to a large pot and cook well over medium-high heat. Shred the chicken after it's cooked through and drain the liquid from the pan.

4. Add the tomatoes to the skillet and let cook for 2-4 minutes. Take off the heat.

5. Add the rice, half of the mozzarella, and half of the parmesan cheese to the pot and stir well.

6. Spoon the mixture into the peppers. Make sure to fill them up. Sprinkle on the remaining cheeses.

7. Pour just a bit of water onto the baking sheet and bake for 35 minutes. Remove and enjoy!

Nutrition Information

(1 pepper/2 half peppers)

Calories: 437, Carbohydrates: 28 g, Fiber: 4 g, Protein: 34 g, Fat: 22 g

Dinner

Roasted Pork Meal (Gluten-Free)

Prep time: 25 minutes

Cook time: 35-45 minutes

Total time: Around 1 hour and 10 minutes

Ingredients

1 ½ pounds of trimmed boneless pork loin

Salt and pepper to taste

5 cloves of garlic

1 pound of potatoes (sweet potatoes work well too)

1 bunch of kale cut into small strips

3 cups of spinach

Lemon juice

2 tablespoons of extra-virgin olive oil

Instructions

1. Preheat your oven to 475 degrees F. Prepare a baking sheet with parchment paper and place the pork on the sheet, seasoning with salt and pepper. Cook for about 25 minutes and let rest.

2. Add the potatoes to a large pot and don't cut them. Add some water to cover the potatoes and bring to a boil. Cover the potatoes and let them simmer for 15 minutes.

3. Add the kale and continue to cook for about three minutes. Add a bit of lemon juice, olive oil, and a little more salt and pepper. Add garlic.

4. Serve all together!

Nutrition Information

(Recipe serves 4)

Calories: 706, Carbohydrates: 22 g, Fiber: 4 g, Protein: 104 g, Fat: 21 g

Black Bean Burgers (Vegan & Gluten-Free)

Prep time: 30 minutes

Cook time: 40 minutes

Total time: 1 hour and 10 minutes

Ingredients

¾ cup of uncooked quinoa

½ of a large chopped red onion

1 cup finely chopped white button mushrooms

Salt and pepper to taste

1 cup of raw, grated beets

1 15-ounce can of low-sodium, drained black beans

1 ½ teaspoons of cumin

¼ teaspoon of paprika

Instructions

1. Cook the quinoa per package instructions. After cooking the quinoa, preheat your oven to 375 degrees F.

2. Sauté the onions in a bit of olive oil in a skillet over medium heat. Add the mushrooms when the onions are translucent and season with salt and pepper. Cook for about 4 more minutes.

3. Remove the pan from heat and add the beans. Mash the mixture a bit—it should look slightly crumbly.

4. Pour the mixture into a large mixing bowl with the quinoa, beets, and remaining ingredients.

5. Chill the mixture in the fridge for about 15 minutes.

6. Prepare a baking sheet with parchment paper and make about 8 patties from the mixture. Place these on the baking sheet before forming patties. Cook for 30 minutes and flip the patties in the middle of the cooking time.

7. Enjoy!

Note: Serve on a whole wheat bun!

Nutrition Information

(For 1 patty)

Calories: 125, Carbohydrates: 17 g, Fiber: 4 g, Protein: 6 g, Fat: 5 g

Chicken N' Pasta Skillet (Gluten-Free)

Prep time: 30 minutes

Cook time: 20 minutes

Total time: 50 minutes

Ingredients

8 ounces of gluten-free pasta

2 tablespoons of extra-virgin olive oil

1 pound of skinless chicken breast

Salt and pepper to taste

4 cloves of minced garlic

½ cup of dry white wine

Lemon juice

10 cups of pre-chopped spinach

4 tablespoons of grated Parmesan cheese

Instructions

1. Cook the pasta according to the package instructions.

2. Bring a separate pan to medium heat and add the oil and chicken. Season with salt and pepper until cooked. Add the garlic and continue cooking for 1-2 minutes. Add the lemon juice and wine and bring the mixture to a nice simmer. Remove from the heat.

3. Add the spinach and pasta. Cover the pot and let the spinach wilt before serving in 4 bowls or plates.

4. Add parmesan cheese to the top and enjoy!

Nutrition Information

(For ¼ of the recipe)

Calories: 335 , Carbohydrates: 25 g, Fiber: 2 g, Protein: 29 g, Fat: 12 g

Squash & Sausage Dinner Casserole (Gluten-Free)

Prep time: 20 minutes

Cook time: 40 minutes

Total time: 1 hour

Ingredients

2 pounds of butternut squash

2 medium pre-chopped white onions

2 cloves of garlic, minced

1 can of drained cannellini beans

1 can of chopped tomatoes

7 ounces of hard sausage

2 tablespoons of extra-virgin olive oil

2 tablespoons of white vinegar

1 cup of vegetable stock

1 tablespoon of honey

Salt and pepper to taste

Instructions

1. Preheat your oven to 360 degrees F.

2. Cut, peel, and cube the squash. Combine onions, beans, garlic, and sausage in a large oven-safe pot and cook on the stovetop until the sausage is slightly browned and the onions appear translucent.

3. Add the remaining ingredients and bring the mixture to a boil.

4. Take the pot off the stove and put it in the oven. Bake for about 30 minutes until the squash appears mushy.

5. Serve!

Nutrition Information

(For ¼ of the recipe)

Calories: 425, Carbohydrates: 48 g, Fiber: 10 g, Protein: 16 g, Fat: 21 g

Vegetarian Risotto (Vegetarian & Gluten-Free)

Prep time: 20 minutes

Cook time: 40 minutes

Total time: About 1 hour

Ingredients

1 cup of short-grain brown rice

½ cup of chopped, dried mushrooms and 1 pound of sliced button mushrooms

2 tablespoons of extra-virgin olive oil

3 cups of pre-cut green beans

½ cup of pre-chopped shallots

½ cup of dry white wine

½ cup of grated parmesan cheese

¼ cup of chopped flat-leaf parsley

Salt and pepper to taste

Instructions

1. Add a few cups of water to a large saucepan and sprinkle in a bit of salt. Add the rice and simmer for about 12-15 minutes. Keep in mind—the rice won't be quite done.
2. Add the ½ cup of mushrooms to a mixing bowl and add three cups of hot water. Let the mushrooms sit for 12-15 minutes and drain, making sure to reserve the liquid.
3. Add half of the olive oil to a separate large skillet and heat over medium. Add the pound of mushrooms and cook until the mushrooms are browned a bit. Add the other mushrooms, green beans, and some salt and pepper, and cook until the green beans are slightly crisp. Add to a separate bowl.
4. Increase the heat in the same pan to medium-high and add the rest of the olive oil. Add the shallots and sauté for 5 minutes. Add the rice and continue cooking for a few more minutes. Season with salt and pepper.
5. Add the wine and cook until it evaporates. Add about ⅓ cup of the mushroom liquid you drained and stir constantly until the liquid is evaporated. Continue with the remaining liquid, waiting until it's evaporated.
6. Pour in the mushroom mixture and cheese. Top with parsley.

Nutrition Information

(For ¼ of the recipe)

Calories: 434 calories, Carbohydrates: 61 g, Fiber: 9 g, Protein: 19 g, Fat: 12 g

Snacks

Salmon, Cream Cheese, and Cucumber Bites (Pescatarian & Gluten-Free)

Prep time: 30 minutes

Cook time: 0 minutes

Total time: 30 minutes

Ingredients

4 ounces of low-fat cream cheese

1 teaspoon of lemon juice

3 tablespoons of chopped chives

1 large cucumber

8 ounces of salmon, pre-cooked and chopped

1 tablespoon of chopped garlic

Salt and pepper to taste

Instructions

1. Remove the cream cheese from the refrigerator and let sit at room temperature for 30 minutes.

2. Combine all ingredients (not the cucumber) in a medium mixing bowl and whisk together.

3. Spoon the cream cheese mixture onto individual slices of cucumber.

4. Serve!

Note: You can make it ahead and refrigerate it for up to two days.

Nutrition Information

(For 1 cucumber slice)

Calories: 22, Carbohydrates: 1 g, Fiber: 1 g, Protein: 2 g, Fat: 2 g

Mozzarella Caprese Skewers (Vegetarian & Gluten-Free)

Prep time: 10 minutes

Cook time: 0 minutes

Total time: 10 minutes

Ingredients

24 cherry tomatoes of different colors (red and yellow are my favorites)

12 mini mozzarella balls

24 leaves of basil

Balsamic vinegar

Salt and pepper to taste

Instructions

1. Collect 12 mini bamboo skewers.

2. Thread 2 basil leaves, 1 mozzarella ball, and 2 tomatoes onto each skewer.

3. Place the skewers on a serving platter and drizzle with some balsamic glaze/balsamic vinegar.

4. Sprinkle with salt and pepper and serve.

Nutrition Information

(For ¼ of the recipe)

Calories: 271, Carbohydrates: 7 g, Fiber: 1 g, Protein: 16 g, Fat: 21 g

Cranberry Bliss Energy Balls (Vegetarian & Gluten-Free)

Prep time: 15 minutes

Cook time: 0 minutes

Total time: 15 minutes

Ingredients

1 cup of gluten-free oats

½ cup of natural almond butter

⅓ cup of natural maple syrup

½ cup of chopped, dried cranberries

4 ounces of white chocolate chips

⅛ teaspoon of vanilla extract

Instructions

1. Combine all ingredients in a stand mixer and mix with the paddle or dough setting until a dough forms.

2. Prepare a baking sheet or dish with parchment paper to prevent the cranberry balls from sticking.

3. Roll the mixture into small balls and refrigerate.

4. Enjoy at your leisure!

Nutrition Information

(For 2 balls; the recipe makes about 24)

Calories: 243, Carbohydrates: 37 g, Fiber: 3 g, Protein: 6 g, Fat: 9 g

Chocolate, Banana, and Walnut Bites (Vegetarian & Gluten-Free)

Prep time: 30 minutes (includes chill time)

Cook time: 10 minutes

Total time: 40 minutes

Ingredients

2 bananas

8 ounces of dark chocolate chips

¼ cup of chopped walnuts or nuts of choice

Instructions

1. Line a baking sheet with parchment paper. Peel the bananas and cut them into 1-inch slides. Place them on the baking sheet and refrigerate for 20 minutes.

2. Add the chocolate to a small microwave-safe bowl and microwave for 20 seconds. Remove and stir. Continue the process until the chocolate is fully melted.

3. Skewer the bananas with popsicle sticks or small skewers and dip them into the chocolate. Don't coat the whole banana slice—just a quarter.

4. Sprinkle on the chopped nuts and refrigerate until serving!

Nutrition Information

(For ¼ of the recipe)

Calories: 266, Carbohydrates: 38 g , Fiber: 2 g, Protein: 5 g, Fat: 14 g

Homemade Beef Jerky (Gluten-Free)

Prep time: 40 minutes

Cook time: 3 hours

Total time: 3 hours and 40 minutes

Ingredients

1 ½ pounds of frozen flank steak

Salt and pepper

1 tablespoon of garlic powder

1 tablespoon chili powder

Instructions

1. Line two baking sheets with parchment paper and preheat the oven to 225 degrees F.

2. Cut the steak against the grain into ¼-inch thick slices. The strips should be about 2 inches long.

3. Place the strips on a plate and let them sit at room temperature for 20 minutes or until they're fully defrosted (up to a few hours). After they're completely defrosted, tenderize them with a meat pounder.

4. Add the strips to a large mixing bowl and add the remaining ingredients. Ensure the strips are well coated.

5. Place the strips on the prepared baking sheets and bake for three hours. Remove from the oven.

6. Let the strips sit for a few minutes before enjoying them!

Nutrition Information

(For ⅛ of the recipe)

Calories: 137, Carbohydrates: 1 g, Fiber: 0 g, Protein: 17 g, Fat: 6 g

Your Post-Menopausal Future

I was discussing menopause with a friend of mine who shared with me that they're "done with it." I asked her what she meant, and she said, "just that, I'm out of it."

I was a little confused. While menopause itself "ends" in a way, the symptoms, and dietary considerations last forever.

It doesn't mean you're old or elderly; remember when you went through puberty? You never thought you'd get the hang of tampons and thought cramps were the *worst*. You got through it, right?

Menopause is like second puberty; it's something to get used to.

Take care of your body. You might be tempted to go on a crash diet or to overload on vitamins: Don't do that just yet.

Try a tailored combination of intermittent fasting and healthy food choices. Remember–balance is key.

Conclusion:

Don't Fear the Future

"I look forward to growing old and wise and audacious."

– Glenda Jackson

Glenda Jackson was right, except for one thing—you're not old. I think the word 'old' is overused. There's nothing old or washed up or undesirable about leaving menopause. You're entering a new stage in your life and that's something to celebrate.

I've given you the tips you need to be successful: We covered the ins and outs of menopause, how to cope with intermittent fasting, and how to fuel your body after a fast. You're not old and you deserve to know the facts.

I spoke to Susan F, a family friend, and writer, who said, "After my periods stopped, I felt relieved. I'd spent my whole life keeping my femininity a secret in a small, locked box. Without that pressure, I feel like I've found the key."

This book is *your* key.

You're not 'less than' after menopause. If anything, you're more than the woman you were before. Femininity isn't intangible; I've given you the skills and tips you need to reclaim your femininity with grace and tact.

I'm not the only success story. Women of all ages can enjoy the joys and benefits of intermittent fasting.

Micia Lopez, in an interview with *Women's Magazine,* said, "I started to fall in love with the idea of intermittent fasting and realized that this, combined with a high-protein diet, was the most beneficial way for me to eat" (Shiffer, 2020).

She told the interviewer, "[She] started cooking pretty much everything. Preparing my food on my own helped me better understand what I was putting into my body" (Shiffer, 2020).

And she's right. Fasting goes beyond the physical; it's a mental transition. When we learn what's going on in our body, we learn how to treat it with respect.

I've said this before, and I'll say it again—there's nothing shameful about menopause. There's no shame in hot flashes, bodily discomfort, or aches and pains. Your body was designed for this process, and instead of beating yourself up about a few extra pounds or a bitter attitude, treat yourself as you would a beloved family member.

The decision to change your life is yours. It's time to make it.

Are you feeling a little more at ease, like someone's in your corner?

Do you feel more comfortable moving through this new life stage?

If you're liking the book so far, please consider helping a fellow

woman and small business owner expand their business! Drop a

review under "Book Review" to help women continue to help women!

Please and Thank You!

Woods Publishing

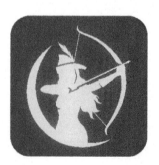

References

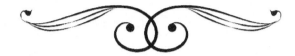

11 facts about body image. (n.d.). DoSomething.org. https://www.dosomething.org/us/facts/11-facts-about-body-image#:~:text=Approximately%2091%25%20of%20women%20are

Bauer-Wu, S. (2018). *How to listen to your body.* Mindful. https://www.mindful.org/how-to-listen-to-your-body/#:~:text=Rest%20for%20a%20few%20moments

Becco, L. (2017). *12 strategies for a safe detox.* Experience Life. https://experiencelife.lifetime.life/article/12-strategies-for-safe-detox/

Boost your metabolism for better health. (n.d.). Beebe Healthcare. https://www.beebehealthcare.org/health-hub/healthy-eating/boost-your-metabolism-better-health#:~:text=The%20benefits%20of%20increasing%20your

Bramlet, K. (2016). *4 things you should know about cleanses, detoxes and fasts.* MD Anderson Cancer Center. https://www.mdanderson.org/publications/focused-on-health/FOH-cleanses-detox-fasts.h10-1590624.html#:~:text=A%20cleanse%20or%20fast%20can

Breenan, D. (2021). *What to know about intermittent fasting for women after 50.* WebMD. https://www.webmd.com/healthy-aging/what-to-know-about-intermittent-fasting-for-women-after-50#:~:text=Research%20shows%20that%20fasting%20can

Breenan, D. (2021). *Psychological benefits of fasting.* WebMD. https://www.webmd.com/diet/psychological-benefits-of-fasting#:~:text=You%20might%20have%20headaches%20or

Brown, L. (n.d.). *Lonny Brown - Holistic health - Adventures in therapeutic fasting.* Sites. Google. https://sites.google.com/site/lonnybrownholistichealth/articles/adventures-in-therapeutic-fasting

Castaneda, R. (2020). *Intermittent fasting: Foods to eat and avoid.* US News & World Report; U.S. News & World Report. https://health.usnews.com/wellness/food/articles/intermittent-fasting-foods-to-eat-and-avoid

CDC. (2016). *CDC - Sleep hygiene tips - Sleep and sleep disorders.* Centers for Disease Control and Prevention. https://www.cdc.gov/sleep/about_sleep/sleep_hygiene.html

Cleveland Clinic. (n.d.). *Postmenopause: Signs, symptoms & what to expect.* Cleveland Clinic. https://my.clevelandclinic.org/health/diseases/21837-postmenopause#:~:text=There%20are%20three%20stages%20of

Coppa, C. (2020). *10 mistakes you can make while intermittent fasting.* EatingWell. https://www.eatingwell.com/article/7676144/mistakes-you-can-make-while-intermittent-fasting/

Eckelkamp, S. (2020). *Intermittent fasting? Here's the right way to break your fast.* Mindbodygreen. https://www.mindbodygreen.com/articles/intermittent-fasting-heres-right-way-to-break-your-fast

Endicott, L. (2019). *Principles of exercise and working out during intermittent fasting.* Simple.life Blog. https://simple.life/blog/exercise-during-intermittent-fasting/

Fletcher, J. (2017). *Menopause bloating: Causes and relief.* Medical news today. https://www.medicalnewstoday.com/articles/319609#when-to-see-a-doctor

Fosu, K. (2022). *3 signs you need a spiritual detox plus ways to do it.* Zora. https://zora.medium.com/3-signs-you-need-a-spiritual-detox-immediately-plus-ways-to-do-it-f8ecc9bbbf98

Francis, N. (2020). *Intermittent fasting and brain health: Efficacy and potential mechanisms of action.* OBM Geriatrics | Intermittent Fasting and Brain Health: Efficacy and Potential Mechanisms of Action. https://www.lidsen.com/journals/geriatrics/geriatrics-04-02-121

Groves, M. (2018). *Menopause diet: How what you eat affects your symptoms.* Healthline. https://www.healthline.com/nutrition/menopause-diet#foods-to-eat

Gudden, J., Arias Vasquez, A., & Bloemendaal, M. (2021). The effects of intermittent fasting on brain and cognitive function. *Nutrients, 13*(9), 3166. https://doi.org/10.3390/nu13093166

Gunasekara, O. (2019). *Growth hormone deficiency & hgh for women.* BodyLogicMD. https://www.bodylogicmd.com/hormones-for-women/growth-hormone/#:~:text=In%20fact%2C%20HGH%20is%20tightly

Gunnars, K. (2019). *10 science-backed reasons to eat more protein.* Healthline. https://www.healthline.com/nutrition/10-reasons-to-eat-more-protein#:~:text=Reduces%20Appetite%20and%20Hunger%20Levels&text=Studies%20show%20that%20protein%20is

Gunners, K. (2020). *Intermittent fasting 101 — The ultimate beginner's guide.* Healthline. https://www.healthline.com/nutrition/intermittent-fasting-guide#_noHeaderPrefixedContent

H, J. (2019). *Working out while fasting is one of the best choices you can make.* Thrive Global. https://medium.com/thrive-global/working-out-while-fasting-is-one-of-the-best-choices-you-can-make-f03453c5067a

Hameed, S. (2022). *Fasting in different religions.* IslamOnline. https://islamonline.net/en/fasting-in-different-religions/Harvard School of Public Health. (2019).

Protein. (n.d.). The Nutrition Source. https://www.hsph.harvard.edu/nutritionsource/what-should-you-eat/protein/

Heffernan, C. (2020). *Guest post: The history of intermittent fasting.* Physical Culture Study. https://physicalculturestudy.com/2020/04/21/guest-post-the-history-of-intermittent-fasting/

History of fasting. (n.d.). Deer Lake Lodge Spa Resort. https://deerlakelodge.com/blog/history-of-fasting

Intermittent fasting. (2019). USNews. https://health.usnews.com/best-diet/intermittent-fasting

Johns Hopkins Medicine. (2021). *9 benefits of yoga.* Hopkins Medicine. https://www.hopkinsmedicine.org/health/wellness-and-prevention/9-benefits-of-yoga

Kelly, L. (2021). *Consumer health: Diabetes and menopause.* Mayo Clinic News Network. https://newsnetwork.mayoclinic.org/discussion/consumer-health-diabetes-and-menopause/#:~:text=The%20hormones%20estrogen%20and%20progesterone

Kubala, J. (2021). *9 potential intermittent fasting side effects.* Healthline. https://www.healthline.com/nutrition/intermittent-fasting-side-effects

Kuta, S. (2021). *Fun ways to exercise: 23 unconventional workout ideas.* Bulletproof. https://www.bulletproof.com/lifestyle/fun-ways-to-exercise/

Leiva, C. (2019). *9 tips for getting enough protein during intermittent fasting.* Insider. https://www.insider.com/getting-protein-while-fasting-2019-3

Lett, R. (2021). *What to eat and drink while intermittent fasting.* Span health. https://www.span.health/blog/what-to-eat-and-drink-while-intermittent-fasting

Link, R. (2017). *13 benefits of yoga that are supported by science.* Healthline. https://www.healthline.com/nutrition/13-benefits-of-yoga

Liu, B., Hutchison, A. T., Thompson, C. H., Lange, K., & Heilbronn, L. K. (2019). Markers of adipose tissue inflammation are transiently elevated during intermittent fasting in women who are overweight or obese. *Obesity Research & Clinical Practice*, 13(4), 408–415. https://doi.org/10.1016/j.orcp.2019.07.001

Mathrick, S. (n.d.). *Fasting - the restorative effects.* Natural Health Mag. https://www.naturalhealthmag.com.au/content/fasting-restorative-effects

Mattson, M. P., Longo, V. D., & Harvie, M. (2017). Impact of intermittent fasting on health and disease processes. *Ageing Research Reviews, 39*, 46–58. https://doi.org/10.1016/j.arr.2016.10.005

Mayo Clinic Staff. (2017). *Menopause: Symptoms and causes.* Mayo Clinic. https://www.mayoclinic.org/diseases-conditions/menopause/symptoms-causes/syc-20353397

Menopause and cancer risk. (2019). Cancer. https://www.cancer.net/navigating-cancer-care/prevention-and-healthy-living/menopause-and-cancer-risk

Menopause and heart disease. (2015). Heart.org. https://www.heart.org/en/health-topics/consumer-healthcare/what-is-cardiovascular-disease/menopause-and-heart-disease

Meserve, C. (2021). *Target the anaerobic heart rate zone and its benefits.* WHOOP. https://www.whoop.com/thelocker/target-anaerobic-heart-rate-zone-benefits/

Morales-Brown, L. (2020). *Intermittent fasting and exercise: How to do it safely.* Medical News Today. https://www.medicalnewstoday.com/articles/intermittent-fasting-and-working-out#why-it-might-not

Daniella, D. (n.d.). *Yoga for menopause: 8 poses for your symptoms.* Moreland OBGYN. https://www.morelandobgyn.com/blog/yoga-for-menopause-8-poses-for-your-menopause-symptoms

National Institute on Aging. (2017). *What is menopause?* National Institute on Aging. https://www.nia.nih.gov/health/what-menopause

National Institutes of Health. (2017). *Vitamin D.* Nih.gov. https://ods.od.nih.gov/factsheets/VitaminD-HealthProfessional/

Owen, A. (2022). *Perimenopause Diet: What to eat for your weight and health.* Join Zoe. https://joinzoe.com/learn/perimenopause-diet

Piersol, B. (2020). *Intermittent fasting and breast cancer: What you need to know.* Memorial Sloan Kettering Cancer Center. https://www.mskcc.org/news/intermittent-fasting-and-breast-cancer-what-you-need-know?amp=

Pullen, C. (2017). *7 ways sleep can help you lose weight.* Healthline Media. https://www.healthline.com/nutrition/sleep-and-weight-loss

Putka, S. (n.d.). *This is your brain on fasts.* Inverse. https://www.inverse.com/mind-body/how-fasting-affects-the-mind-and-the-body

Semeco, A. (2020). *20 simple ways to fall asleep fast.* Healthline. https://www.healthline.com/nutrition/ways-to-fall-asleep#1.-Lower-the-temperature

Shields, A. (2020). *What actually happens to your body during a fast, hour by hour?* Mindbodygreen. https://www.mindbodygreen.com/articles/what-happens-when-you-fast

Shiffer, E. (2020). *"When I started this weightlifting routine, I dropped 30 lbs. in 2 months and got my shape back."* Women's Health. https://www.womenshealthmag.com/weight-loss/a31144156/intermittent-fasting-high-protein-diet-weight-loss-success-story/

Sisson, M. (2020). *How to exercise while fasting.* Mark's Daily Apple. https://www.marksdailyapple.com/how-to-exercise-while-fasting/

Stangl, K. (2022). *The 4 things I wish I had known before I started intermittent fasting.* The Spruce Eats. https://www.thespruceeats.com/what-to-know-before-intermittent-fasting-5216293

Summer, J. (2021). *The benefits of intermittent fasting for sleep.* Sleep Foundation. https://www.sleepfoundation.org/physical-health/intermittent-fasting-sleep#:~:text=How%20Does%20Intermittent%20Fasting%20Affect

Szalay, J. (2015). *What is fiber?* Live Science. https://www.livescience.com/51998-dietary-fiber.html

The slow start to fasting. (2022). Ciccone Family Chiropractic and Wellness Center. https://cicconechiro.com/the-slow-start-to-fasting/

The yoga-heart connection. (2019). Johns Hopkins Medicine. https://www.hopkinsmedicine.org/health/wellness-and-prevention/the-yoga-heart-connection

Visioli, F., Mucignat-Caretta, C., Anile, F., & Panaite, S.-A. (2022). Traditional and medical applications of fasting. *Nutrients,* 14(3), 433. https://doi.org/10.3390/nu14030433

Vitamin D. (2012). The Nutrition Source. https://www.hsph.harvard.edu/nutritionsource/vitamin-d/#:~:text=It%20is%20a%20fat%2Dsoluble

Wdowik, M. (2017). *The long, strange history of dieting fads.* Source. https://source.colostate.edu/the-long-strange-history-of-dieting-fads/

Williams, C. (2018). *How intermittent fasting affects your metabolism.* Cooking Light. https://www.cookinglight.com/healthy-living/healthy-habits/how-fasting-affects-metabolism

Winona Editorial Team, & Green. (2022). *HRT health benefits for intermittent fasting and menopause.* Winona Wellness. https://bywinona.com/journal/intermittent-fasting-and-menopause

Wolff, C. (2016). *10 ways to exercise without realizing it, according to fitness experts.* Bustle. https://www.bustle.com/articles/184536-10-ways-to-exercise-without-realizing-it-according-to-fitness-experts

Working out while intermittent fasting. (n.d.). Atkins. https://www.atkins.com/how-it-works/library/articles/6-things-to-know-about-intermittent-fasting-and-working-out

Zhao, Y., Jia, M., Chen, W., & Liu, Z. (2022). The neuroprotective effects of intermittent fasting on brain aging and neurodegenerative diseases via regulating mitochondrial function. *Free Radical Biology and Medicine*, 182, 206–218. https://doi.org/10.1016/j.freeradbiomed.2022.02.021

Made in the USA
Las Vegas, NV
13 February 2024

85691068R00096